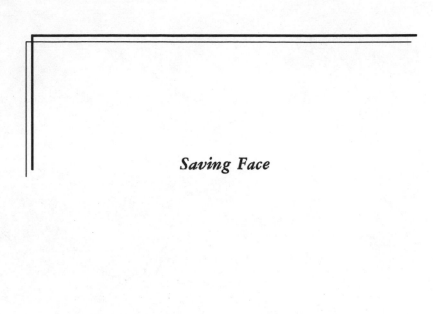

Saving Face

SAVING FACE

Nelson Lee Novick, M.D.

*A Dermatologist's
Practical Guide to
Maintaining a Healthier
and Younger Looking Face*

Franklin Watts New York 1986

ILLUSTRATIONS BY ANNE CANEVARI GREEN

Library of Congress Cataloging-in-Publication Data

Novick, Nelson Lee.
Saving face.

Includes index.
1. Face—Care and hygiene. 2. Skin—Care and
hygiene. 3. Face—Aging. 4. Skin—Aging. 5. Beauty,
Personal. I. Title. [DNLM: 1. Aging—popular works.
2. Comestics—popular works. 3. Dermatology—popular
works. WR 100 N943s]
RL87.N68   1986   616.5   86-15920
ISBN 0-531-15022-4

*To my wife Meryl, without whose understanding,
patience and support this book would not have
been possible; and to my sons Yonathan, Yoel,
Ariel and Daniel, without whose presence in my
world no accomplishment would seem worthwhile.*

Contents

PART II
WHAT YOUR DOCTOR
CAN DO FOR YOU

With thanks to my office manager, Barbara Jerabek, whose comments, suggestions and technical assistance were invaluable in the preparation of this book.

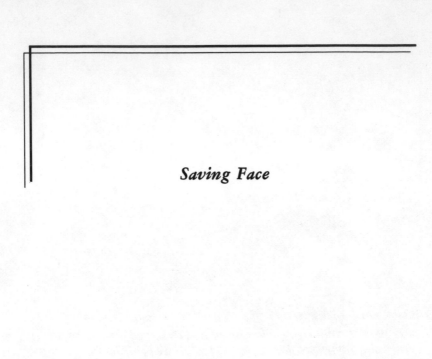

Saving Face

Preface

Jeff is forty. Every morning he drags himself out of bed, squints at himself in the bathroom mirror, closely examines his puffy eyes, carefully notes every wrinkle on his face, checks to see whether he's developed any new crow's feet at the corners of his lids, and then curses the reflection in the mirror. He then stumbles back to the bed, stands over his wife Betty, pulls back on his puffy lids, stretches out his wrinkle lines, and asks, "Wouldn't I look much better if I had this puffiness here, and those wrinkles there, removed, like this?"

Betty is thirty. Every morning, right after her husband leaves for work, she stands by her three-way facial mirror in the bathroom, checks to see whether the wrinkle lines around her mouth have deepened since the day before, looks carefully to see if any pimples have cropped up on her face and neck, repeatedly examines the bridge of her nose to reconsider whether she should have that small bump removed, and then pats the underside of her jaw, while making strange faces as she does her stretching exercises to shrink her double chin. She finally proceeds to cover every imperfection she can possibly find with an array of new "youth restoring" and "revitalizing" cosmetics that she has recently purchased. Finally, she leaves the bathroom, totally disapproving the recent condition of her face and what Father Time has been doing to her.

Jeff and Betty are two patients in my private practice. While most people probably do not go through such an elaborate morning ritual, most of us, as we grow older, do take stock of the changes in our skin and hair. Because we can so easily examine our own faces in the mirror, facial aging can be particularly distressing to us. For most of us, aging facial skin has become our enemy—an enemy to be fought in any way we can.

At one time, particularly within the ancient Eastern cultures, the outward signs of aging were considered signs of wisdom, experience, and distinction. Over the past several centuries, however, particularly in Western culture, this philosophy slowly changed. Nowadays, like Ponce de Leon four centuries ago, we search for the fountain of youth.

Today a youthful appearance is highly prized and much sought after. Consumers spend many millions of dollars annually on skin care products that claim to do everything from growing hair on bald heads, to shrinking dilated pores, eliminating wrinkles, and fading age spots; and fortunes are spent by advertisers to convince people that their products do just those things. Some of these products, bearing the flashiest packaging Madison Avenue can manage, and presented very alluringly in the media and magazines, may cost as much as eighty dollars for half an ounce. Given all the technical and catchy jargon that is used in these advertisements, how are you, the consumer, to know what to believe and what to buy?

Medical science, too, has kept pace with the growing patient demand to look and feel younger. Much research and study have been devoted to the problems and questions related to aging of the skin. Great advances in cosmetic, dermatologic, and plastic surgery offer the opportunity to have wrinkles smoothed, scars removed, noses fixed, sagging eyelids tightened, and most recently, fat sucked from the jowls and from under the chin. While the results of these procedures are for the most part gratifying, the procedures frequently cost a great deal, require absence from work, and usually entail some operative or postoperative discomfort.

The array of offerings to help you keep looking young, then, is dizzying. Some of them are good, some useless, and some bad. How are you to know what to choose? It would seem a medical education is necessary just to make the right choices. This book is intended to help you make better choices. Based upon current scientific principles and my own clinical experience with thousands of patients, it is a practical guide intended to lead you through the maze of conflicting claims, information, and misinformation.

In Part 1, "*What You Can Do for Yourself,*" I have translated into nontechnical terms current information about skin and the basic changes that occur in facial skin aging. Here, too, are some very essential facts about skin care products and cosmetics and how to choose them according to your specific needs. I have made every effort to separate fact from fancy about scalp, hair, and skin care, in order to give you the necessary background against which to judge what you see and hear in advertisements. In sum, Part 1 provides you with the essentials for knowing what you can *realistically* do for yourself.

A common complaint about doctors these days is that they haven't enough time to talk with their patients. Frankly, most busy doctors find it all but impossible to spend the time they would like explaining all the details of your particular medical or surgical treatment. However, this information is crucial. Without it, it is difficult to intelligently decide whether you even wish to try a certain medication or have a certain procedure done. Without it, you cannot assess cost-effectiveness or long-term benefits. You can't even properly plan your own business or social schedules.

Therefore, in Part 2, "*What Your Doctor Can Do for You,*" the various kinds of medical and surgical procedures available for treating aging facial skin, as well as other conditions, are explained. You will learn what each of these procedures entails and what you can realistically hope to gain from them.

Naturally, owing to rapid scientific and technological progress, new products and new procedures are constantly being developed. Nevertheless, the basic information provided in this book will continue to serve you by providing you with essential information and guidelines. This information will enable you to better understand your doctor's medical or surgical recommendations and make you a more active participant in the decision-making process. Only in this way will you be truly able to make the most of your looks, your time, and your money.

Throughout the book, I have mentioned, by brand name, a variety of cosmetics and drugs for various conditions. These products are ones with which I have had considerable personal experience and have found to be consistently effective. *I am not, however, endorsing any product or products or any generic substance.* The products I've mentioned are by no means the only products available for dealing with the conditions discussed, nor does exclusion from my list of recommended skin care items imply that a particular product is not necessarily equally effective. Where some products have been found worthless, I clearly say so. I do suggest, however, that you consult your dermatologist if you have any questions about the value or efficacy of a specific drug or cosmetic. Finally, given the nature of this book, descriptions and explanations of medical therapies and surgical procedures must be addressed to the general concerns of a wide audience. Should you have any particular concerns about any form of therapy described in this book, you should of course ask your doctor. Finally, this book is not intended to be relied upon as a substitute for the advice of, or consultation with, your doctor.

Some Facts about
Skin and Skin Aging

In *Saving Face*, I have written a lot about the kinds of products you can buy or methods that you or your doctor can use to help you to obtain a healthier, more youthful appearance. To better understand the rationale for these products and procedures, you need to be aware of a few basic facts about skin, particularly aging skin.

Normal, healthy skin is divided into three basic layers, each with different functions: the *epidermis, dermis,* and *subcutis.* (Figure 1 is a schematic cross-sectional diagram of normal skin.) The epidermis is composed of a relatively thin, but tough, protective, top layer of dead skin cells, the *stratum corneum,* sometimes called the horny layer. The horny layer is made up largely of the protein *keratin.* Below the horny layer, you find a second, thicker layer of living and rapidly growing epidermal cells called *squamous cells.* New skin cells are constantly being produced in the bottommost row of squamous cells, the *basal layer.* From there, newly "born" cells move upward through the squamous layer toward the skin surface, supplying your skin with fresh cells every day. At the same time new cells are being made, dead cells from the horny layer are constantly being shed. Contrary to what Madison Avenue would like you to believe, your skin is incapable of "eating" or "drinking in" most chem-

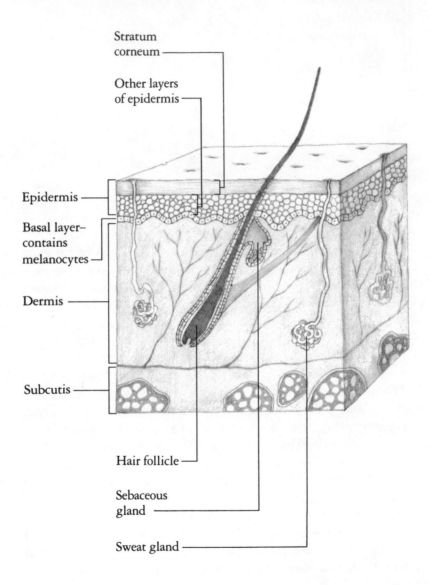

Stratum corneum

Other layers of epidermis

Epidermis

Basal layer– contains melanocytes

Dermis

Subcutis

Hair follicle

Sebaceous gland

Sweat gland

FIGURE 1.
Schematic diagram of normal skin (cross section)

icals applied to it. Few substances applied to the skin are truly able to penetrate the epidermis.

Pigment cells or *melanocytes* are responsible for producing the skin pigment, *melanin*, and are found scattered through the *basal layer* of the epidermis. Melanin imparts a brownish hue to your skin and hair. In any individual the exact amount of melanin and its distribution is genetically determined. The precise manner in which melanin is distributed through the skin is a major determinant of mankind's racial differences. Melanin production increases during periods of increased sun exposure and functions to protect your skin from the damaging effects of the sun's ultraviolet radiation.

Below the epidermis lies the dermis, the supporting layer of the skin. This extremely important layer contains nutrient-delivering blood vessels, sensitive nerve endings, and the much-talked-about supporting and stretching fibrous proteins of your skin, collagen and elastin. Largely unsubstantiated claims for replenishing or rejuvenating these fibers, particularly the collagen, through the application of "secret," "Old World," or "European" cream and ointment formulations continue to be the subject of much advertising hype. In reality, the only significant nutrition supplied to your skin is delivered from *below*, through your dermal blood vessels.

Below the dermis is the fatty layer, or subcutis, which serves as a cushion and energy source for the skin. Hair follicles, oil glands, and the sweat glands course through all the layers of your skin down to the fat. The oil glands, or *sebaceous glands*, secrete oil into the hair follicles to which they are attached. The oil then rises to the surface along your hair shafts and exits through your pores. Oil gland secretion is responsible for locking in the skin's natural moisture and preventing dryness. Contrary to popular belief, the oil itself does not lubricate or moisten the skin, but merely serves as a barrier to retain the moisture that is already in your skin cells. The sweat glands of the face, the *eccrine glands*, produce an odorless secretion composed largely of water that exits to the surface through its own pores and functions to regulate your body temperature through evaporation.

You are probably familiar with the various outward manifestations of facial aging—facial contour changes, increases in the facial prominences, recession of teeth, and diminution in the vertical height of the mouth. Characteristically, the natural action lines of the face deepen to become wrinkle lines. The skin becomes lax and begins to sag into folds and pouches. Loss of color occurs both in the skin and hair.

What actually happens to your skin as you age? That question has been the subject of intensive scientific investigation, particularly during the past few years. Not all the answers are known, but certain useful facts have been established. Briefly, as skin ages, it tends to become thinner, produce fewer cells, and grow more slowly. The protective horny layer becomes less effective. The epidermis becomes thinner, particularly where it joins with the dermis. New cells are produced more slowly, and older or damaged cells are repaired less effectively. Individual cells that were once uniform in size become variable. The number of pigment-producing melanocytes decreases.

The dermis also becomes thinner and retains less water. Blood vessels become fewer, and nerve endings may become abnormal, leading to altered or diminished sensation. Sweat and oil gland activity decreases, and glandular secretions may decrease dramatically with advanced age, leading to dryness and itching. Collagen and elastin fibers become more rigid and inelastic, and the skin begins to wrinkle and sag. Facial skin wrinkles and sags, not as some believe, due to loss of tone in the facial muscles, but rather due to changes in the supportive proteins in the dermis, primarily collagen. This is why, contrary to popular belief, isometric exercises will not eliminate wrinkles and sags. It simply is not a muscle problem but a skin problem.

Years of overexposure to the sun exaggerates and accelerates one's hereditary natural aging process. Finally, with advancing age, skin also becomes more susceptible to the formation of a variety of both benign and malignant skin tumors.

Aging affects other areas of your skin. In the subcutis there is a loss and redistribution of fat. Loss of fatty tissue in the wrong places tends to emphasize sagging skin. Scalp hair becomes thinner, sparser, and grays; eventually it whitens in color. At the same time, unwanted hairs may become thicker and darker in the ears and nose and on the upper lip.

The purpose of this brief chapter is not to paint a bleak picture of skin aging, but simply to provide you with the sort of knowledge that should make you better able to judge any advice or claims made by beauticians, cosmeticians, and skin and hair care product manufacturers—and also better able to understand the rationale for the products and procedures discussed in *Saving Face*.

PART I

WHAT YOU CAN DO FOR YOURSELF

1

Choosing the Right
Facial Cleanser

Today, the sheer number of print advertisements and television commercials urging you to buy this lotion or that soap which is guaranteed to rejuvenate your skin and make you look twenty-five years old again is formidable. Beautiful young models, exotic-sounding ingredients, and fantastic claims about using ancient Eastern or Old World "secret formulas" to create their cleansing preparations are the manufacturers' ploys to lure you into buying their frequently expensive products so that you can "let product X" make this happen for you. What are you supposed to believe? What is the truth about soaps and cleansing creams? What can they actually do, and which ones are really best?

SOAPS

Soap is simply any skin cleanser made from the salts of animal or vegetable fats. Coconut oil or palm kernel oil is frequently added to make a soap lather better. This then is the formula of your so-called basic toilet soap. Toilet soaps generally tend to be slightly alkaline. Cleaning with plain toilet soap and water removes most environmental and natural skin surface substances, such as dirt, cosmetics, oils, bacteria, dead skin cells, and sweat. Except for so-called "soapless soaps," which contain synthetic detergents, most kinds of soaps advertised differ only in addition of other, often non-essential, ingredients.

IVORY soap is probably the industry standard for plain basic soap. For people with normal skin, IVORY will usually do the job of cleaning efficiently and inexpensively. But for people with very sensitive skin or other skin conditions, it may be too drying and irritating. If you have problem skin, you may find the following kinds of cleansing products useful.

SUPERFATTED SOAPS

Superfatted soaps contain extra amounts of oils and fats, such as lanolin, olive oil, cocoa butter, neutral fats, or cold cream. The inclusion of oily ingredients is supposed to prevent the usual tendency of soap to dry out your skin. Recent evidence lends some support to this claim. Superfatted soaps attempt to perform the delicate balancing act of removing grease and grime from your skin (a drying effect) while depositing a cold cream or fat in its place (a moisturizing effect). It is actually a testimony to modern cosmetic chemistry that a product can be composed of ingredients that have two directly opposite tasks and still remain useful. Nevertheless, for the most part, superfatted soaps do pretty much what they are designed to do. (These soaps apparently do a good enough job to cause some people to complain about feeling "greasy" or "unclean" after using them. For these people, I usually recommend a soapless soap, which will be discussed later.) I have found DOVE soap, PURPOSE soap, BASIS soap, and OILATUM soap all to be satisfactory superfatted soaps.

TRANSPARENT SOAPS

Transparent soaps, like superfatted soaps, contain a somewhat higher fat content, usually in the form of increased castor oil or resin. They are, therefore, useful for cleansing dry or sensitive skin. Other ingredients such as glycerin, alcohol, and sugar are added to give these soaps their transparency and soft consistency. Unfortunately, transparent soaps tend to lather poorly and melt easily in soap dishes, properties that occasion frequent complaints. However, their useful life *can* be prolonged by removing them from the soap dish and drying them off. No proof exists that transparent soaps are actually any better for sensitive skin than superfatted soaps. Again, personal preference should be the deciding factor. NEUTROGENA soap is a popular form of transparent soap.

SOAPLESS SOAPS

Sometimes called detergent soaps or bars, soapless soaps contain synthetic soaps (detergents) made from petroleum derivatives. Cosmetic chemists have attempted to alter synthetic detergent soaps to make them less alkaline, less irritating to your skin, and capable of lathering better. I still find a good lather difficult to obtain with these soaps. Nevertheless, they seem to satisfactorily clean the skin. As a rule, I have no objection to the use of soapless soaps for people with sensitive skin. I usually suggest LOWILA cake to my patients who dislike the greasy afterfeel of some of the superfatted soaps.

At this point, I must emphasize that almost any soap or detergent cleanser, no matter how good it is, can still be somewhat drying to your skin. In order to be an effective skin cleaning agent, a soap or detergent must be able to degrease your skin oils and debris; by its very nature, then, it must be somewhat drying. You can minimize a soap or detergent's tendency to be drying by being less physically abusive to your skin when you clean it. In other words, when you wash, don't superscrub your skin. Whenever possible, apply a good moisturizer after you gently dry your face.

CLEANSING CREAMS
AND LOTIONS

Cleansing creams are basically variations of the formula for cold cream to which other ingredients have been added. These additional ingredients are supposed to impart special properties to the cleansing cream or to lend elegance to the product.

Cleansing creams are usually recommended for people with dry, sensitive skin. They are meant to be applied to the skin and then wiped off with a soft tissue. Because the proportions of the basic ingredients have been somewhat altered, cleansing creams are generally lighter and less oily than cold cream; nevertheless, like cold cream, they usually leave a greasy film on your skin. For this reason they generally make poor cleansers. Oily or acne-prone skin may even be made worse by their use. Further, to eliminate any sticky residue or greasy, unclean feeling, many people follow the cleansing cream ritual with either the use of a toning solution or a vigorous soap and water cleansing. Unfortunately, this defeats the very purpose of a cleansing cream. Its lubricating benefits are essentially nullified by the drying effects of the toner or soap cleansing.

Yet cleansing creams can be useful in a few specific situations. You may find them helpful in removing heavy waterproof makeups, water-fast masking cosmetic products, and stage makeup. However, after the cosmetics are removed, you should follow up with a gentle soap and water cleansing, using the kinds of soaps mentioned earlier. With the exception of these situations, I generally do not recommend the routine use of cleansing creams.

Liquefying creams contain the same basic ingredients as cleansing creams, except that the oils and waxes contained in these products have been formulated to melt upon contact with your skin. However, there seems to be no particular cleansing advantages to using a liquefying cream instead of a cleansing cream.

Cleansing lotions have the same basic ingredients as cleansing creams, except that more water has been added. Lotions, in general, have somewhat less drag on your skin and can be wiped off with a tissue a little more easily than cleansing creams. Otherwise, they share the same pros and cons of cleansing creams.

WASHABLE CREAMS
AND LOTIONS

Washable creams or lotions (soapless cleansers) contain many of the same basic ingredients as cleansing creams. However, varying amounts of soap or detergents have been added to these products to enhance their oil- and grease-removing abilities. These products are intended to be rinsed off in plain water, rather than wiped off with a tissue; hence the designation washable creams. Washable lotions simply contain more water than washable creams, but are otherwise about the same.

Washable creams and lotions can be helpful if you have excessively dry skin. As a rule, most people using washable creams do not feel as clean as they do after a soap and water cleansing. On the other hand, if you have excessively dry, sensitive skin, it is better for your skin if you don't try to get it "squeaky clean"; the effort may simply irritate it.

For patients with dry and sensitive skin I often recommend that they alternate the use of gentle soap and water cleansing with the use of washable creams or lotions. You might, for example, use soap and water to clean your face in the morning and use a washable lotion at night. For sensitive skin this is often much less irritating than washing twice daily with soap and water and can be an especially helpful measure in the wintertime when skin chapping is a common problem for many people. If your skin still remains dry after a routine such as this, you may find it better to use the washable cleansing cream or lotion by itself or to alternate its use with soap every other day.

Summertime can be a difficult season for sensitive skin;

excessive chlorine exposure from pool swimming or overexposure to the sun can be very drying. Here again, washable cleansing creams or lotions used by themselves or in alternation with soap and water may be more gentle to your skin than the routine use of soap and water.

By incorporating a washable cleansing cream or lotion into your skin cleaning routines, you have greater latitude to tailor those routines to meet your changing needs throughout the year. I find CETAPHIL lotion and PHRESH 3.5 lotion excellent choices in this category.

SOAPS TO AVOID

Fruit, Vegetable, and Herbal Soaps

Fruit, vegetable, and herbal soaps are soaps or detergents to which various "natural" ingredients have been added. The special ingredients are supposed to make you think *health*, and *the great outdoors*, about which you hear so much these days. However, the basic working ingredients of these kinds of soaps are much the same as those contained in any other soap. The fruit, vegetable, or herbal additives are strained, sterilized, and treated with alcohol and preservatives as part of the manufacturing process, and are then mixed with fragrances and coloring in order to make them resemble, once again, the real thing. Even if there were some proven benefits to washing your skin with fruits or vegetables in the first place (which there isn't), the nature of the soap manufacturing process eliminates them. What remains of the fruits, vegetables, or herbals in these soaps after the manufacturing process only superficially resembles any product of the fresh, great outdoors. These soaps serve no especially useful function and are certainly not worth the often considerably higher prices charged for them. The bottom line: Fruit, vegetable, and herbal soaps really do little for your skin, but much to lighten your wallet.

Abrasive Soaps

Abrasive soaps are cleansers that contain tiny particles that serve to mildly abrade your skin. They are essentially intended to rub off the very top surface only and are usually recommended for tough cleaning jobs. For most people, however, they can be too harsh and too drying. I sometimes recommend them for periodic use to people who complain of exceptionally *oily* skin. On skin with acne or certain other types of inflammation, abrasive soaps can frequently be quite irritating and should be used only upon the advice of a physician.

Medicated Soaps

Medicated soaps are cleansers to which a variety of different medicinals such as sulfur, salicylic acid, benzoyl peroxide, or antiseptics have been added. These additives are ones that have been found to be effective for treating certain conditions such as infection, acne, or eczema when incorporated into topical creams and lotions. However, there is no hard evidence that when these same ingredients are combined with soap, they have any effect at all. It has been found that in order to have some beneficial effects on your skin, medicated ingredients must remain in contact with it long enough to begin work. Soaps, which are lathered up and rinsed off almost immediately, do not permit the necessary contact time for the medication in them to do much good. As a result, medicated soaps generally offer no particular advantage over regular toilet soaps and are frequently more drying. In general, avoid them.

Deodorant Soaps

Deodorant soaps, also called antibacterial soaps, have little place in facial skin care. Skin odor is the result of bacterial breakdown of the secretions of specialized sweat glands called *apo-*

crine glands. Deodorant soaps are basically plain soaps to which antibacterial additives have been incorporated for suppressing the growth of the odor-producing bacteria on your skin. These soaps may also contain perfumes for masking odor. Since your face does not contain apocrine glands, antibacterial soaps are unnecessary for facial skin cleansing. They tend to be overly drying. Nevertheless, they *can* be excellent body soaps. If you wish to continue using a deodorant soap for your body, choose a milder soap for your face.

In summary, if you have dry, sensitive skin, you would do well to choose one of the superfatted soaps, soapless soaps, or washable lotions. Which brand you will ultimately prefer will most likely be determined by that product's basic appeal to you. Basic appeal simply means how well you believe a particular product cleans, how your skin feels during and after its use, whether you like its fragrance, bar size, and shape, and—if it's an expensive soap—how long it survives in your soap dish. Pass up soaps that contain exotic ingredients, and be skeptical of almost-too-good-to-be-true claims made for the facial cleanser; they usually are not true. Consider your budget. Some very good soaps may be conveniently purchased in the supermarket for almost one-third the price of similar soaps sold in a pharmacy.

Most important, though you need soap to clean your skin, keep in mind that no soap is really good for the skin. They cannot make you younger looking or wrinkle-free, as some manufacturers would like you to believe. On the other hand, knowing that you should choose the gentlest, least drying, least irritating cleanser is an important step to healthier skin.

Now that you know more about which soaps to choose, I have some general guidelines for best using them. Naturally, these may need to be modified depending upon your individual circumstances and needs. These guidelines are primarily meant for people who have basically normal or naturally dry or sensitive skin, or whose recreational activities expose them to a lot of sun, wind, and weather. If you have a specific skin condition, I urge you to consult your dermatologist.

Most of you tend to wash yourselves too frequently and too vigorously. For many, overzealous scrubbing arises out of the misconception that in order to make your skin look better, you must scrub away the bad stuff. The reality is quite the contrary. Generally, you should avoid washing your face with soap and water more than once or at most twice a day. Depending upon the season and weather you may need to wash your face even less.

In wintertime, when you are exposed to the drying effects of wind and lowered humidity outdoors, and lowered humidity from central heating indoors, you may need to reduce facewashing to once daily. I usually recommend that you wash with plain water in the morning to refresh yourself and reserve the soap and water cleansing for the nighttime to help with makeup removal. In the summertime, you may find that overexposure to the sun, chlorine, and prolonged exposure to air-conditioning (which lowers indoor humidity), can be just as drying to your skin as winter conditions. Again, you may need to reduce soap and water cleansing to once daily.

If a psychological need to feel clean overpowers you and you feel you absolutely *must* wash your face frequently in order to feel clean, splash on plain water only. While you should not use soap at these times, you may use cleansing lotions. If you find that washing your face even just once a day leaves it too dry, you may be better off skipping soap altogether and routinely using a cleansing cream or lotion. While you may not feel as clean as you would after using soap and water, your skin will be smoother, less dry, and more comfortable.

Follow each facewash with the use of a good moisturizer (Chapter 2). As you will learn in Chapter 2, however, no amount of moisturizer can adequately make up for an over-zealous scrubbing with soap and water.

Even though most of you probably enjoy the relaxing feeling of washing with hot water, you should avoid it. The combined effects of hot water, soap or detergent, and vigorous massaging of the skin can overly degrease your skin and open the way to dryness, chapping, itching, and irritation. Instead, be sure to rinse with plenty of plain, *lukewarm* water to remove all traces of soap residue. If you live in a "hard" water area, use a synthetic detergent soap. The calcium and magnesium mineral deposits in hard water react with regular soaps to leave a thick residue on your skin (and sink basin, for that matter) that is difficult to rinse away, and thus can lead to irritation. Synthetic detergent soaps are specifically made to leave little or no residue in hard water and are easily rinsed off.

If you follow these few simple guidelines for washing your face, your skin will look clean, feel clean, and remain moist, smoother, and healthier.

2
Fighting Dryness—
The Truth
about Moisturizers

In my practice, many of the most frequently asked questions relate to the subject of moisturizers. Which is the best moisturizer? Can they really keep me younger looking, prevent wrinkles, remove wrinkles, or slow down skin aging? Questions such as these reflect the enormous influence of advertising in the manufacturers' efforts to convince you that each of them has got the secret cream or lotion to work miracles for your face. However, before answering these questions, I feel that some basic information about how your skin keeps itself lubricated and what makes it become dry will be instructive.

Naturally moist, smooth, and supple skin results from sufficient amounts of three major elements: water, oil, and special chemicals called *natural moisturizing factors.* Under ordinary circumstances, 95 percent of each of our cells is made up of water. The water content of your skin cells is the major determinant of how moist and supple your skin is. If for any reason your skin cells lose water and begin to dry out, you will have problems with your skin. Wrinkles, which, contrary to a popular misconception, are *not* caused by dryness, may be accentuated by it. Dry skin can also make you more prone to scaling, cracking, irritation, eczema, and infection.

Yet, because of the skin's importance, nature has provided ways to keep it from drying out. To minimize water loss, your sebaceous glands (oil glands) manufacture and secrete oils onto the surface of your skin where they act as a natural oil barrier to prevent water loss through evaporation. Your natural oils do not themselves moisturize your skin; they merely help to hold on to the water you already have in your skin. Natural moisturizing factors are another means utilized by your skin to maintain its water balance. Natural moisturizing factors are substances normally present on your skin that have a special attraction for water; they are able to absorb water from the atmosphere and hold it to your skin. Perhaps now you can better understand why I was so emphatic in Chapter 1 about advising you *not* to over-scrub with hot water and soap, which can wash away your skin's natural oil barrier and natural moisturizing substances and leave you dried out and sensitive.

Ideally, any commercial moisturizers and lubricating routines for your face should be directed to restoring and maintaining the normal water balance of your skin. Perhaps in hope of increasing their product's consumer appeal or distinguishing their product from their competitor's, some manufacturers and advertisers have added confusion to the subject of moisturizers by claiming that their products contain *lubricants* or *emollients*. To eliminate any mystique from these terms, a few simple definitions are in order. A moisturizer is an ingredient that can make your skin more supple or less dry-feeling, and promote smoothness. A lubricant is an ingredient that increases the silkiness of your skin, promotes a smooth feeling, and makes a product more spreadable. An emollient is an ingredient or product used to smooth and soften the skin. Basically, you can see that these three terms mean about the same thing, and for all practical purposes can be used interchangeably. However, the bottom line, no matter what you read or hear, is that moisturizers, lubricants, and emollients promote smoothness and softness of the skin, and that's all.

It is important to realize that the true function of most moisturizing creams or lotions currently available is *not* to add any moisture to your skin, but to prevent the loss of water from your skin through evaporation, or to lock on to water from the atmosphere. Despite what some manufacturers would like you to believe, moisturizers are *not* absorbed into your skin; nor can they do a lot of other things that have been claimed for them, such as shrinking pores, preventing wrinkles, or rejuvenating skin.

Most moisturizers are composed of the same basic ingredients: water, oils, wax, emulsifers (to keep the oil and water mixed), fragrance, and preservatives. They generally come in the form of creams or lotions; the latter are simply moisturizing creams to which more water has been added.

Moisturizing products may differ in the proportions of oil and water as well as the specific oils contained in them. (The types of oils most frequently found in moisturizing preparations are discussed later in this chapter.) So-called "oil-free" moisturizers, as their name implies, contain less oil and more water. If you carefully examine product labels, however, you will find that even so-called oil-free products do contain some oil. Without it, they would likely have no moisturizing effects at all.

A quick and useful way to obtain a good idea of how oily or watery a particular product might be is to rub a little of it onto the back of your hand. A product with more water than oil will, in a matter of seconds, begin to cool the back of your hand because of the evaporation of its water. A product with more oil than water will not do this; in fact, the back of your hand may even feel slightly warmer because of the coating of oil on your skin.

Depending upon your particular skin care needs, you should choose a product that has the right combination of oil and water. I generally recommend moisturizing lotions rather than creams for the face. Many people find creams too thick and greasy to routinely use on their faces and prefer the feel of a lotion, which is generally less occlusive and more easily applied. However, if you do have exceptionally dry or flaking skin, I would suggest that you use a cream moisturizer, at least until your skin has improved considerably. You may then switch back to a lotion if you wish. I also usually advise creams for those whose work or recreation requires considerable outdoor exposure to cold, wind, low humidity, or excessive sunlight.

Many wild claims are made by advertisers for the benefits of the particular oils contained in their products. Some claim that their oils can rejuvenate the skin. Others claim that theirs can slow the aging process or eliminate wrinkles. In addition, you will find moisturizers containing various kinds of exotic ingredients, which are often associated with inflated claims for their remarkable skin-saving properties—and even more inflated prices·for the moisturizers that contain them. In the following sections, I discuss in greater detail the four major types of oils found in most moisturizing creams and lotions, as well as the various kinds of special ingredients that are most frequently added to supposedly enhance a moisturizer's effectiveness.

ANIMAL FATS

Lanolin, mink oil, turtle oil, and codfish oil are all examples of animal fats. These oils, particularly lanolin, which is derived from the oil glands of sheep, closely resemble human oil gland (sebaceous gland) secretions. Hydrous wool fat is one common form of lanolin, but there are many other derivatives of lanolin. Owing to their resemblance to your normal skin oils, moisturizers containing animal fat usually interfere the least with the normal functioning of your skin, and for these reasons make excellent moisturizers. Mink and turtle oils, while comparable to lanolin, do not offer any additional moisturizing advantages, despite claims to the contrary. They can add considerably to the price of the product containing them, however. In the case of turtle oil, some advertisers subtly try to play up the notion that since turtles live so long, their oils must have some age-retarding properties. This is, of course, nonsense (though it would be wonderful if we could find the answers to the turtle's longevity).

MINERAL OILS

This category includes regular mineral oils and petroleum derivatives. Petrolatum, or petroleum jelly as it is commonly called, has been used for over one hundred years, and it is still found in many cosmetics and topical medications. Petrolatum is excellent for preventing the loss of moisture from your skin and protecting it against environmental irritations. In fact, petrolatum is still considered the paradigm of moisturizers against whose effectiveness all others are judged. Mineral oil does about the same job. Some people with extremely dry or cracking facial skin, who dislike fragrance-containing creams or lotions, will find the use of mineral oil or petroleum jelly products very satisfactory for moisturizing. An allergy to petrolatum is about as rare as a hen's tooth; for those of you who have trouble finding a moisturizer to which you are not sensitive, you would do well to apply plain petroleum jelly to your face at night. For most people, however, the greasiness and oiliness of these products, and the fact that they cannot be easily applied or removed from the skin, make them less esthetically appealing.

VEGETABLE OILS

Olive oil, safflower, corn, wheat germ, palm kernel, apricot, sesame, and all other nut oils are vegetable oils that have been incorporated into moisturizers. In general, they make satisfactory moisturizers. However, they are usually not as effective as the animal fats or mineral oils. While a higher proportion of polyunsaturated vegetable oils in our diet seems to have a beneficial role in the prevention of heart disease, vegetable oils appear to have no special beneficial effects when applied to the skin. Nevertheless, manufacturers have gotten good mileage from the implied association.

EXOTIC AND OTHER
EXTRA-ADDED INGREDIENTS

The ingredients discussed in the following sections are the ones that usually are the center of much advertising hype. They are also the ingredients often responsible for the fantastically high prices of some creams and lotions for which you may pay up to eighty dollars a half-ounce.

Vitamin E

Vitamin E, or as it is sometimes found in the list of cosmetic ingredients, tocopheryl acetate, has become increasingly popular. People are taking large amounts by mouth for a variety of reasons, ranging from cancer prevention to increasing sex drive. They are also applying it directly to their skin, either by breaking open vitamin E capsules and applying the liquid, or using commercial moisturizing lotions and creams containing tocapheryl. Vitamin E has been touted for skin rejuvenation and for speeding wound heading. Unfortunately, none of these claims has been scientifically substantiated. Yet one thing *is* for certain: vitamin E cannot pass through the topmost layer of your skin. Therefore, it is unlikely that it can do anything at all when applied to the skin except add to the price of the product. A caveat is in order here: A number of my patients who have used vitamin E tablets for various reasons have developed severe allergies to it and required anti-allergy treatments.

Collagen, Proteins, and Amino Acids

Collagen, other proteins, and amino acids—but most especially the collagen—are advertised as special ingredients that possess the power to make your skin look younger. Amino acids are the building blocks of proteins. Proteins, in turn, make up the structural building blocks of your body, and collagen is one particularly important form of structural protein.

Collagen fibers make up our connective tissue, cartilage, and bone. As I mentioned earlier, changes in collagen fibers with the passage of time contribute to wrinkling and aging of the skin. Under normal circumstances, collagen and other proteins are constantly being broken down in our skin while new collagen and other proteins are being produced to replace them. The body uses the amino acids in our diet to do this. Collagen or other proteins applied to the skin in the form of moisturizing creams or lotions cannot be absorbed through the skin because of the size of the molecules. Contrary to what the advertisements say, your skin *cannot* eat up the collagen; hence, the amino acids, collagen, or other proteins in certain moisturizing creams and lotions are only as effective as the oils they contain. Because there are so many expensive preparations containing collagen out there, it bears repeating: the collagen in these preparations simply cannot get down to the portion of skin where it is needed.

It is extremely important that you do not confuse the collagen found in moisturizing preparations with the injectable form of collagen (ZYDERM collagen), that is successfully used for the correction of wrinkles, pock marks, and scars. That form of collagen is *injected* by a physician through a very fine needle into the uppermost layer of your skin. It is placed exactly where it is needed and it is not purported or intended to be eaten up or absorbed by your skin. (This is discussed in greater detail in Chapter 13.)

Hormones

The majority of moisturizers with hormones contain small amounts of the female hormones estrogen and progesterone. Manufacturers of hormone-containing moisturizers claim that their products are capable of reversing the skin aging process in several ways: thickening of the topmost layer of the skin, regeneration of aged or sundamaged skin, and stimulation of the skin's own natural oil gland secretion. *No* conclusive evidence exists that these hormone preparations can do any of these things for you. They may, however, attract and hold on to water, and in this way may contribute somewhat to smoother, more supple skin. In my opinion, the possible advantages of hormone-containing moisturizers do not justify their additional cost and I therefore seldom recommend them.

Placental extracts have also been incorporated into moisturizers for their hormone and vitamin contents. In any of these preparations, you often don't know exactly how much of anything you are actually getting. The implied desirability of moisturizing products containing placental extract is that since the placenta is known to be a source of nourishment for the developing embryo, it can somehow maintain or impart youthfulness to your skin. As I have already said, the overall value of putting hormones into moisturizers is equivocal at best. With this in mind, if you wish to try a hormone-containing moisturizer, you should at least choose one where the exact ingredients are specified on the label.

Natural Moisturizing Factors

Earlier in the chapter I mentioned that your skin naturally contains certain substances called natural moisturizing factors that attract and hold on to water at the skin surface. Some manufacturers have attempted to incorporate a number of these substances into their products to improve their moisturizing potential. Urea compounds, and more recently lactic acid, glycolic acid, and lecithin compounds (a phospholid), are increasingly being used. Since these substances also help to loosen scales, they frequently give your skin a smoother, softer feeling. I have found the moisturizers containing these ingredients to be highly satisfactory for even my problem patients. Most people especially appreciate the fact that these preparations usually do not leave a greasy film on their skin.

In general, if you have extremely dry or sensitive skin you should use those products containing high concentrations of the ingredients. If your skin is normal or only mildly dry, stick to the moisturizers with the lower concentrations. I have found this class of moisturizers to be quite effective, particularly the products containing urea. As an added plus, many of them have been tested and found to be nonacnegenic, and therefore you may use them even if you have acne. They can be particularly helpful in countering the drying effects of many of the anti-acne topical medications.

In addition to the natural moisturizing substances, these products, like other moisturizers, usually contain some form of oil as well, to provide barrier protection and to prevent water evaporation. Although the jury is not yet in on all these products, I have been very impressed with their usefulness. Of particular help are: AQUACARE/HP lotion, CARMOL-10 LOTION, COMPLEX-15 lotion, and LAC-HYDRIN LOTION (currently by prescription only).

Unusual or Exotic Additives

In trying to decide which moisturizer is best for you, you may come across claims for the almost "magic" rejuvenating properties of algae, aloe vera juice, eggs, honey, or vegetable extracts. Algae are simple plant life, like seaweed or pond scum. Aloe vera juice is an extract of the aloe plant leaf and is nearly 100 percent water. Neither of these ingredients has been shown to add anything to the moisturizing value of the products that contain them. Any benefits that you might find are undoubtedly the result of the oils that are also contained in the products.

Even though the exotic or special ingredients seem to command all the advertising fanfare, if you carefully examine the labels of the moisturizers containing them, you will usually find these ingredients listed near the end. According to product labeling regulations, those ingredients that are in the highest concentrations in a product are listed first. Invariably, you will find the product's moisturizing oils listed first on the ingredient label; it is really from these oils, rather than from the relatively small amounts of exotic additives, that those products derive their moisturizing capabilities.

Eggs, milk, and honey are three other favorite ingredients for which fantastic advertising claims have been made. Eggs may be quite nourishing to developing embryos, milk very nourishing for infants, and honey quite nourishing for bees, but none of them do anything in particular for your skin. In fact, all these ingredients have been known to cause allergic reactions in allergy-prone individuals. Furthermore, although *lecithin* is one of the skin's natural moisturizing factors, the lecithin in eggs is not in a form that is particularly useful when you apply it to your skin. Your skin cannot "eat or drink up" any of these foods or substances. My recommendation is to avoid products containing these ingredients! They usually do nothing for your skin, and their cost is frequently high.

No matter what you hear or read, the major function of moisturizers is to provide your skin with protection from excessive dryness by preventing water loss and holding on to water. Moisturizers cannot restore youth, rejuvenate your skin, or dissolve your wrinkles. To make things easier for yourself, follow these simple guidelines when you shop for moisturizers.

1. Remember that inexpensive moisturizers generally do as good a job as expensive ones and be skeptical of any wild promises.
2. Within the confines of your personal taste and budget, choose a moisturizer that feels comfortable on your skin and, most importantly, *use it* as often as possible, particularly after you wash.

Even though moisturizers can't really make your skin younger, when used properly, they can at least help to "baby" it.

3

*The Sun—A Wolf
in Sheep's Clothing*

The subject of this chapter is one that I have repeatedly found
to have the power to stir up a hornet's nest of emotions with
my patients whenever I bring it up. Since the 1920s, tans have
been associated with good health and the good life. Like fresh
air, warm breezes, and fresh milk, the sun is a symbol of nature,
of all things wholesome and naturally good for you. But is the
sun really good for you? Is that golden tan many of you yearn
and strive for really healthy, or is it actually a signal that your
skin is being over-stressed by the sun? Just how much sun exposure is too much?

Without question, sun exposure is not without certain benefits. Exposing your skin to the ultraviolet rays of the sun increases your own natural production of an essential vitamin,
vitamin D. In addition, I'm sure many of you will agree that
being outdoors under a warm sun can be a psychologically uplifting, frequently exhilarating experience. Finally, there is no
denying that a golden suntan can temporarily make you look
youthful and healthy while it hides blotchy skin and a host of
other ills.

Unfortunately, science has learned that the sun is really a
wolf in sheep's clothing. In the first place, the vitamin D issue
has been overplayed. In fact, all the sun-induced vitamin D
synthesis that you need can be gotten from one fifteen-minute

period of sun exposure to an area of your skin no larger than the size of the back of your hand. Besides, in the Western world, where diet is adequate, most of us get enough vitamin D from the foods we eat. Anything beyond that can only hurt your skin, not help your body. Furthermore, it is pretty firmly established that chronic overexposure to the sun can result in three types of sun damage: sunburn, premature aging, and skin cancers. Because of this, I frequently tell my patients that in the scheme of nature it seems that plants and vegetables were meant to be out in the sun, but not people.

HARMFUL EFFECTS
OF SUN EXPOSURE

Those of you who have gotten sunburned can really appreciate what that condition is all about. Depending upon the severity of the burn, a sunburn reaction can run the gamut from painful reddening of your skin to severe blistering. The height of the reaction usually occurs within six to twenty-four hours after overexposure to the sun. In severe cases of sunburn, victims may even require hospitalization. In most cases, however, simple lotions, compresses, or baths and occasionally prescription oral medication are all that are required to treat it. But that may not be the end of the story. Individual episodes of sunburn, particularly during childhood and adolescence, have been linked to the development of malignant melanoma, a potentially life-threatening form of skin cancer about which you will learn more in Chapter 17.

The sun is responsible for premature aging. Each of us has a built-in genetic time clock for aging, and each of our organs ages at a different rate. Recent articles in the medical literature now suggest that those signs of skin aging that we have always attributed to the simple fact of getting older or to genetic inheritance in large measure may actually be the product of years of accumulated sun damage. The sun can hasten wrinkling and thinning of your skin, and cause the appearance or accentuation of blotchy brownish or tannish discolorations and "broken" blood vessels. The extreme case of sun damage is the "weather-beaten" (actually sun-beaten) nape of a sailor's neck.

There exists an enormous body of evidence linking the accumulated effects of years of sun exposure to the formation of skin cancers. More than 90 percent of all skin cancers occur on the sun-exposed areas of the body—the face, neck, forearms, hands, legs, and to a lesser extent the upper back. Basal cell skin cancer, squamous cell skin cancer, and melanoma are the three main types of skin cancers (all of which are discussed in Chapter 17).

Twenty years of "frying" yourself in the sun can leave you looking fifteen to twenty years older than you really are. You can easily do a little test to prove this to yourself. For most of you, there is one area of your body that has just about never seen the light of day—your buttocks. Carefully compare it to the skin of your face, V of your neck, or arms. Compare these areas for texture, the presence of age spots or of heaped up brown spots (called *keratoses*). Look for "broken" blood vessels, wrinkling, sagging, loss of smoothness, leatheriness, or blotchy discolorations of red, yellow, or gray. You will probably be quite surprised to find that your buttocks actually look better and more youthful than your face and neck. If natural aging was the sole factor in skin aging, every area of your skin, exposed and non-exposed, would age evenly. Without question, the *sun is the culprit*.

To sun lovers, this kind of information is anathema. Unfortunately, many respond by pooh-poohing, denying, or rationalizing. Some take a "Why worry now?" attitude, assuring themselves that a cure for skin and skin cancers is right around the corner. Others insist that they feel healthier when they are in the sun so, despite what I say, it must really be healthful. One of my patients, a noted world traveler, television celebrity, and ardent sun lover, summed up his feelings: "The sun is the way of the world!" Understandably, many people express concern that they will not be able to pursue their accustomed outdoor recreational or exercise activities that they feel they need to remain healthy in other ways.

And it does seem to fly in the face of reason that a golden brown, healthy-looking tan can really be bad for you. Nevertheless, it is! That golden tan that so many of you crave reflects the fact that the ultraviolet light from the sun has penetrated through at least the upper layer of your skin, to which your skin has responded by producing and redistributing more of its melanin pigment in order to minimize further damage to itself from the ultraviolet rays. In other words, *suntan* really means *skin damage.* If you want "just a little tan," it means that you will have just a little damage. A deep tan means a lot of damage has taken place. Unfortunately, long after your tan fades, the damage to your skin will remain. The effects of a lot of "little tans" accumulate over the years. Suntanning is like slapping your cheeks. It may temporarily add color to your face and make you look healthier, but in fact it is a trauma to your skin.

Since this book is all about maintaining a younger, healthier-looking face, you must come to terms with the fact that the sun is not your skin's best friend, but its arch foe, as much as you may dislike hearing it.

But since the sun is here to stay, and since most of us can't seem to stand the thought of ever completely giving it up, the next section of this chapter will describe some ways that you can peacefully coexist with the sun. In order to do this you first need some more facts about the sun.

ULTRAVIOLET RADIATION

In addition to visible light from the sun, the sun sends out invisible light rays called *ultraviolet radiation.* About one-twentieth of the rays that we receive on earth are ultraviolet rays. Ultraviolet A (UVA) and ultraviolet B (UVB) are two important types of ultraviolet light that are transmitted through our atmosphere. A third, strong type of ultraviolet light from the sun, ultraviolet C (UVC), is filtered out by our atmosphere and is of no consequence.

Damage from ultraviolet radiation is responsible for suntans, sunburns, premature aging, and skin cancers. The total amount of this ultraviolet radiation that you receive on any occasion depends upon a number of factors: the season of the year, the time of day, weather conditions, how close you are to the equator, and how much and what type of protective clothing you wear.

Where you live in the world determines which times of the year the sun's rays will be most intense. For the northern latitudes, the time of the year when the earth tilts toward the sun extends from mid-April to mid-October. In places south of the equator, such as Australia, the hottest times of the year are between mid-October through mid-April. At or near the equator, the sun will be intense all year long. If you live anywhere in the continental United States, you require the most sun protection from mid-spring through mid-autumn.

Where you live also determines the amount of sun's rays you receive per hour. A person living, for example, in Canada, receives less ultraviolet light hour-for-hour of exposure than a person living closer to the equator, say, in Texas. In fact, the Texan would quite likely receive as much as two times the amount of the sun's rays per hour. People living or vacationing in high altitudes are also more likely to burn because the thinner atmosphere of mountainous regions less effectively blocks out the sun's rays.

The time of day is another very important factor and should be considered when you plan your outdoor activities. No matter where you live, the sun's rays are always strongest between the hours of 10 A.M. and 3 P.M. because the rays are more direct at those times, and you are most likely to sunburn during those hours. Chances of sunburning are much less before 10 A.M. and after 3 P.M., when the sun is no longer overhead and the angle of its rays is more slanted.

Inclement weather conditions can give you a very false sense of security when you are outdoors. Most people think that a partly cloudy or foggy day means a day without sunburn. In fact, as much as 80 percent of the sun's rays may be transmitted through fog and clouds and can still cause a severe sunburn. On windy, but sunny days your risk of sunburning is usually increased, simply because it is usually cooler and more comfortable—and therefore possible to remain out in the sun longer. Cool breezes do *not* in any way diminish the ultraviolet radiation you receive. Surprisingly, they may even enhance the untoward effects of the sun. Hot days, too, can increase your risk of sun damage by potentiating the effects of the ultraviolet radiation. High humidity can also do this. Another important fact to remember (especially for those of you who love to ski and thought that you were treating your skin better by vacationing in Aspen rather than Fort Lauderdale) is that you can get very sunburned while skiing. Fresh snow is capable of reflecting back at you as much as 80 percent of the sun's rays.

Beach umbrellas and certain types of clothing can give you a false sense of security outdoors. It is a common misconception that all kinds of clothing afford the same kind of protection and that light colored clothing is better. In fact, the color of your clothing actually makes little difference; the fabric and weave do. Cotton fabrics provide superior protection from sunlight, and tightly woven fabrics afford better protection than loose weaves. Most clothing is at least somewhat protective. Be aware, however, that wet, clinging clothing can more effectively transmit ultraviolet light to your skin.

If you enjoy sitting outdoors under beach umbrellas, boardwalks, or shady trees, you should be aware that between 60 to 80 percent of the sun's rays may be reflected onto you from the surrounding sand and water. For that matter, sunlight is even transmitted through the water. If you think that you are fully protected from the sun by keeping most of your body submerged, you are mistaken. Ultraviolet light can get through to you.

Even if you aren't a sun worshiper, you still have to exercise "sun sense" whenever you are outdoors. At a recent dermatology symposium on the sun and its ill effects, it was emphasized that many people, and many doctors for that matter, associate sun-damaged skin only with beach-loving sun worshipers. These people certainly are at risk, but we tend to forget that during warm sunny months, many of us expose ourselves to a good deal of sun just by enjoying our favorite outdoor activities. Even a simple twenty-minute daytime stroll a few times a week can add up to a lot of unintentional sun exposure. And, this incidental kind of sun exposure on unprotected skin over several years can be quite damaging.

In my practice, I have a number of patients who grew up in the sunbelt areas of the United States, but claim to have always disliked the sun and shunned sunbathing. Nevertheless, I found in many of them the same kinds of sun damage that one sees in those who are dedicated sun lovers. Thus, considerable damage can be caused by even incidental, *unintentional* sun exposure when proper precautions are not taken. These patients were exposed to too much sun just by going about their normal business in a sunny climate; while they didn't seek out the sun, the sun found them anyway. And since they didn't realize just how much sun they were actually getting, they also never made any effort to protect themselves either by wearing proper protective clothing or using sunscreens.

SUNLAMPS AND
TANNING PARLORS

No discussion of ultraviolet radiation would be complete without some reference to the use of sunlamps and tanning parlors. Everything you have just read about the dangers of excessive UVA and UVB radiation from the sun applies equally to the ultraviolet radiation obtained from artificial sources. In addition, recent evidence suggests that some artificial ultraviolet light sources may also generate UVC, a highly potent skin cancer-inducing type of ultraviolet radiation. The very fact that sunlamps are so accessible and easy to use makes them potentially more dangerous than natural sunlight. After all, on a cold, snowy day, you can't expose yourself needlessly to the sun in order to keep your tan, but you can very easily sit under a sunlamp. Their potential for overuse constitutes a real danger. I do not recommend them. However, if you insist upon using them, do so infrequently, not daily.

It is estimated that there are between one thousand and two thousand tanning salons in the United States today. Most tanning parlors use ultraviolet light B, the kind most associated with sunburn and skin cancer formation. Some tanning salons entice their customers by offering ultraviolet A (popular in Europe). These salons claim that they can tan you safely with UVA, with little risk of causing either sunburn or skin cancers. Even if this were so, recent evidence seems to indicate that UVA may be the major culprit associated with premature aging of your skin. For these reasons, I strongly advise you against frequenting any tanning salons, either of the UVA or UVB kinds.

SKIN TYPES

Having answered the *what, where, when,* and *whys* of sun exposure, I would like to turn to the *who.* Everyone seems to know somebody who loved to bake in the sun, always had a golden tan, and now doesn't seem to have a wrinkle. Obviously, not everyone is equally susceptible to sun damage. *Who* is most likely to run into problems from the sun? Dermatologists classify individual sun susceptibility according to six skin types.

> Type I   — Always burns; never tans—i.e., extremely sensitive
> Type II — Always burns; sometimes tans—i.e., very sensitive

Type III — Sometimes tans; sometimes burns—i.e., sensitive

Type IV — Always tans; sometimes burns—i.e., minimally sensitive

Type V — Always tans; never burns—i.e., not sensitive

Type VI — Negroid skin—i.e., not sensitive

Ethnic background is a very important determinant of your skin type. For example, people of Scotch-Irish (Celtic) origin are usually Type I people of North European descent, such as Germans and Scandinavians, and are generally either Types I or II. As a rule of thumb, light, fair-haired, light-eyed, and fair-complected people of any ethnic background usually fall into Types I or II. People of Mediterranean origin, such as Italians, Greeks, Spaniards, etc., generally are Types IV and V, and people of Hispanic or Oriental background are usually Type V. However, variations in skin type do exist between individuals of the same ethnic or racial backgrounds, depending largely upon how much ethnic dilution took place in that particular group. That is, not all blacks necessarily have type VI skin; some with lighter skin may have Type III or IX skin and will show the same degree of sun susceptibility as any white person of the same skin type.

SUN SENSE

By this time you may feel flooded with facts, a little confused, perhaps disappointed, and maybe even a little angry. You now know that the sun is basically no good for you, but you may not be quite sure exactly what you're supposed to do about it, and you've definitely decided that, no matter what, you're not going to become a hermit and go off and live in a cave somewhere. The following guidelines should help you continue to enjoy the sunny outdoors and still do much to maintain a younger and healthier-looking face.

Sunscreens

To prevent incidental, unintentional sun exposure between April and mid-October (northern hemisphere), you should routinely apply a sunscreen preparation to your skin every day. If you make it as much a habit as combing your hair or brushing your teeth, you will be less likely to forget to do it. I suggest you use the sunscreen as an undermakeup moisturizer instead of your usual moisturizer. More and more manufacturers are routinely including sunscreens in their moisturizing products. Ideally, you should apply a sunscreen in an air-conditioned room, at least twenty minutes before going out.

Many different types of sunscreen preparations are available in all price ranges. Some offer complete protection, while others claim to allow you to tan, not burn. The following section should help you to choose the right product for you.

Sunscreen preparations vary widely in their sun-protective abilities. *Sunblocks* are products designed to provide you with 100 percent protection from the sun. That means no suntan, no sun damage. These products contain opaque, physical barriers, such as titanium dioxide or zinc oxide. Such products are meant to be applied only to limited areas of the body, such as the nose. The white cream that you frequently see on the noses of lifeguards is zinc oxide ointment. The drawbacks to these preparations are that they are meant to be used only on limited areas of the skin and they are too thick and too esthetically displeasing for most people's taste. RV-PAQUE ointment contains a flesh-toned pigment to make it more cosmetically acceptable.

Mineral oil, baby oil, cocoa butter, and coconut oil preparations do nothing more than simply lubricate your skin. Moisturizing your skin *after* sun exposure is a good idea, since sun exposure does tend to dry out your skin. However, these preparations as sunscreens provide absolutely *no protection whatever* from the harmful rays of the sun. As a matter of fact, mineral oil may actually be responsible for focusing the sun's rays and making matters worse. (If your skin needs to be moisturized, follow the suggestions given in Chapter 2 for choosing and using an appropriate moisturizer.) Iodine, which stains the skin a brownish color, has been added to some mineral oil preparations; however, like the mineral oil, it does nothing to protect your skin.

By classifying sunscreen preparations as drugs, the Food and Drug Administration made the task of choosing an effective sunscreen easier. Each manufacturer is required to label its sunscreen product with an SPF (Sun Protection Factor) number. SPF numbers generally range from 2 to 23. The higher the SPF, the greater the sun protection it provides. Here's how it actually works. If you are the kind of person who would sunburn after just fifteen minutes in the sun, and if you use an SPF 15 product, it would take approximately 225 minutes or three and three-quarters hours (15×15 minutes) for you to burn.

Several chemical ingredients are commonly found in the majority of sunscreens. These are paraaminobenzoic acid (PABA) and derivatives of PABA called PABA esters (e.g., padimate A and padimate O), benzophenones, cinnamates. Some preparations contain a combination of two or more of these ingredients. Because of the variety of effective ingredients, should you develop an allergy to any one of them, you can switch to a chemically unrelated product and can still expect excellent sunscreen protection. I generally advise patients to use products with SPF numbers 15 or better because they provide the maximum protection. No matter how high the SPF number, you can still expect to get some tan, especially if you remain out in the sun the entire day. Physical barrier products and appropriate clothing are the only ways to ensure complete protection from the sun.

The particular brand of sunscreen you use matters little as long as you choose the right SPF number for your skin type and *as long as you use it.* In general, my patients have expressed satisfaction with the following SPF 15 sunscreens: TISCREEN,

SOLBAR PF, ECRAN, SOLBAR PLUS, and TOTAL ECLIPSE. Your choice will depend largely upon your budget and personal preference for such things as feel and fragrance.

Many sunscreens are either alcohol-based or cream-based. Alcohol-based sunscreens tend to be somewhat drying to your skin. Cream bases naturally tend to be moisturizing. For those of you with oily skin, I recommend the alcohol base. (These products may sting when first applied.) For most people, however, I recommend the creamy, moisturizing sunscreens. They go on easily, especially when applied in a cool, dry room, and they are useful for counteracting the somewhat drying tendency of the sun on your skin.

If you have light eyes, a fair complexion, and have Type I or II skin, or are someone who already shows wrinkles, I would strongly advise you to use a sunscreen of SPF 15 or better. If you have had a history of skin cancer, you most certainly should. If you have no prior history of sun-related skin problems and you have Type III skin, you may, for example, use sunscreen products in the range of SPF 8 to 15. If you have Type IV skin, you can use products that are labeled SPF 4 to 8. If you have Type V or VI skin, you probably don't require any sunscreen at all, but this depends on exactly how dark your natural skin tone is.

Sensible Rules for Tanning

If, after all you have just read, you still can't resist the urge to go out and get a golden tan, you should at least develop your tan gradually and try not to sunburn yourself inadvertently. If you have sun-sensitive skin (Types I or II), your first exposure should be no longer than fifteen to twenty minutes on the first day. You may start with twenty to twenty-five minutes if you are a Type III, twenty-five to thirty minutes if you are a Type IV, and so on. If, for example, you have Type II skin and you choose to use a sunscreen product with an SPF 6 or 8 (though I recommend SPF 15) and apply it thoroughly, you can remain outdoors six to eight times longer on your first exposure, approximately one and a half to two hours (SPF 6 or 8 × 15 minutes).

On each day of the first week of sun exposure, you may increase your exposure time by one-third of the previous day's time. By the end of the first week, your skin will have thickened enough and will have produced enough melanin pigment to provide you with additional protection from sunburn. The best time of day for working on your tan is before 10 A.M. or after 4 P.M., especially if you are beginning your tan at the height of the summer season or if you are on winter holiday in an intensely sunny climate.

Artificial Tanning Agents

The use of an artificial tanning preparation is a safer way to add color to your skin, without having to expose yourself to the potential dangers of the sun. Chemical tanning agents and bronzers are two popular types of artificial tanning formulations. These products should not be confused with sunscreens. They do not protect you from the sun; they merely give you the appearance of having been out in the sun.

Chemical tanning agents rely upon the harmless chemical reaction of a dye, usually dihydroxyacetone (DHA), with your skin. Chemical tanning dyes generally need to be reapplied every few days. A major drawback: If you don't like the color you get (and sometimes it can appear quite artificial), it normally takes several days for you to lose your chemical "tan." It takes three to four days until the chemically dyed outer layer of your skin is shed naturally or in the course of routine skin cleansing. To prevent a possibly embarrassing situation, I suggest you do a small patch test to see how you like the result. If you are satisfied with the color of the test site, you can then apply the chemical tanner to the rest of your face and body. No matter how dark they make your skin, chemical tanning agents offer no protection from the sun. You must still protect yourself with a real sunscreen when you go outdoors.

Bronzers are a second kind of safe, artificial "tanning" product. They contain a pigment that is merely deposited on your skin; no true chemical reaction takes place between the pigment and your skin. The obvious advantage of bronzers is that they may be washed off immediately if you don't like the resulting "tan." The disadvantage, of course, is that if you do like it, you must reapply the bronzer after each washing. Bronzers, like chemical tanning agents, do not confer any significant protection from the sun's rays. Once again, regardless of how "tan" you appear, should you wish to go out in the sun, you must take the same precautions as you would otherwise have needed.

Pre-Sunbathing Tan Promoters

Recently, a new type of tanning product was introduced which, when applied for several days prior to sunbathing, is supposed to promote the development of a quicker tan when you go out into the sun. The combination of ingredients in these formulations is supposed to stimulate your skin to increase its own melanin production. The medical community is still awaiting the publication of hard scientific data to support these claims.

Tan-promoting agents raise another, even more important issue than whether or not they truly work to promote tanning. Products like these, as well as others that make sunbathing more attractive to consumers, serve to encourage people to go out and get a tan. Given the proven dangers of sun exposure to your skin, it might be reasonable for the FDA to require that such products carry a label on their boxes as cigarettes do— "WARNING: The Surgeon General has determined that sunbathing is hazardous to your skin."

4

Choosing the Right
Cosmetics for
Beauty and Camouflage

Cosmetics, according to their legal definition, are products manufactured for the sole purpose of making you look better. By contrast, topically applied medications are defined as products that are intended to have an effect on either the structure or function of your skin. By these definitions, drugs are subject to stringent Food and Drug Administration regulation, while cosmetics escape it—although the FDA does insist that ingredients contained in a cosmetic be listed on its label to warn consumers who may be allergic to some or all of them. Specific information on fragrances or flavorings contained in cosmetics need not be listed on the label, however. Moreover, unlike topical medications, the FDA does not require efficacy testing for cosmetics. Cosmetic manufacturers are required only to have performed sufficient testing on their products to assure their general safety. Ultimately, the responsibility for success and satisfaction with any particular cosmetic falls largely to you, the consumer. You should always read carefully all cosmetic labelling and directions before buying and using any cosmetic.

Cosmetics are big business. Roughly $1.5 billion are spent annually on skin care cosmetics (mostly by women), and this figure is expected to continue to climb at a rate of about 15 percent per year. Different brands of cosmetics intended for the same purposes, and whose active ingredients may be quite similar or even identical, may range in price from pennies per ounce to eighty dollars or more per ounce. What guides you to select one brand over another often remains largely a matter of your individual preferences for fragrance, color, feel, attractive or eye-catching packaging, or simply successful advertising hype. My purpose in this chapter is not to tell you which specific cosmetic brands to buy, but to give you some useful information to bear in mind when you do buy. I have also provided explanations about some of the major ingredients found in many cosmetics. Finally, the special masking makeups specifically developed for camouflaging a wide variety of scars and other disfiguring skin conditions are discussed.

Cosmetic chemistry is a highly complex field, and even a brief glance at almost any cosmetic ingredient label is usually enough to make you feel overwhelmed and confused. To make matters worse, the same cosmetic ingredient may be listed on one product label by its trade name, on another by its generic name or chemical name, and on still another by its common name. For example, carbomer, a common gel-forming ingredient found in many products, also goes by the names of carbopol or carboxyvinyl polymer. This, of course, makes it especially difficult for you to compare the cosmetic ingredients of one product with those of another.

In general, product ingredient labels can be confusing and sometimes even misleading. At the very least, you should be aware that product ingredients are listed on package labels in the order of their relative amounts in the product. In other words, even without knowing specifically how much of a particular ingredient a product contains, you will at least know that it contains more of those ingredients listed first on the label than those listed last. The Cosmetic Toiletry and Fragrance Association publishes the *CTFA Cosmetic Ingredient Dictionary*, which for the professional at least helps to unravel some of the confusion. For practical purposes, Table 1 lists, according to their main functions, many of the basic ingredients found in a wide variety of cosmetic creams and lotions. I have listed them by

TABLE 1

COMMON COSMETIC INGREDIENTS BY FUNCTION

Emollients

Butyl stearate
Caprylic/capric triglyceride
Castor oil
Cetearyl alcohol
Cetyl alcohol
Diisopropyl adipate
Glycerin
Glyceryl monostearate
Isopropyl myristate
Isopropyl palmitate
Lanolin
Lanolin alcohol
Lanolin, hydrogenated
Mineral oil
Petrolatum
Polyethylene glycols
Polyoxethylene lauryl ether
Polyoxypropylene 15 stearyl ether
Propylene glycol stearate
Silicone
Squalane
Stearic acid
Stearyl alcohol
Vegetable oils

Humectants

Glycerin
Propylene glycol
Sorbitol solution

Solvents

Alcohol
Diisopropyl adipate
Glycerin
1,2,6-hexanetriol
Isopropyl myristate
Polyoxypropylene 15 stearyl ether
Propylene carbonate
Propylene glycol

Emulsifying agents (Surfactants)

Amphoteric-9
Carbomer
Cetearyl alcohol (and) ceteareth-20
Cholesterol
Disodium monooleamidosulfosuccinate
Emulsifying wax, NF
Lanolin
Lanolin alcohol (Laureths)
Lanolin, hydrogenated
Lecithin
Polyethylene glycol 1000 monocetyl ether

Polyoxyl 40 stearate
Polysorbates
Sodium laureth sulfate
Sodium lauryl sulfate
Sorbitan esters
Stearic acid
Tea stearate
Trolamine

*Emulsion stabilizers
and viscosity builders*

Carbomer
Cetearyl alcohol
Cetyl alcohol
Glyceryl monostearate
Paraffin
Polyethylene glycols
Propylene glycol stearate
Stearyl alcohol

*Preservatives, antioxidants,
and chemical stabilizers*

Alcohol
Benzyl alcohol
Butylated hydroxyanisole (BHA)
Butylated hydroxytoluene (BHT)
Chlorocresol
Citric acid

Edetate disodium
EDTA
Imidazolidinyl urea
Parabens
Phenyl mercuric acetate
Potassium sorbate
Propyl gallate
Propylene glycol
Quarternium-15
Sodium bisulfite
Sorbic acid
Tocopherol (Vitamin E)

*Thickening, stiffening,
and suspending agents*

Beeswax
Carbomer
Cellulose gums
Cetyl esters wax
Dextrin
Polyethylene
Xanthan gum

Gellants

Carbomer
Carboxymethyl cellulose
Hydroxymethyl cellulose
Methyl cellulose

their most commonly used names. This list, of course, is not complete, but it should dispel some of the mystery and confusion inherent in product labeling. (A more complete list is beyond the scope of this book. In addition, many of the chemicals listed frequently have more than one function.)

COMMON COSMETIC INGREDIENTS AND THEIR FUNCTIONS

No matter how complicated or exotic-sounding the names of particular cosmetic ingredients may be, they usually serve one or more of several basic functions—as emollients, emulsifying agents, stabilizers, thickeners, gellants, solvents, humectants, or preservatives. In general, very few of the ingredients that you see on a product label are the active ingredients for which you may be buying the product. Most ingredients are put there to prevent spoilage, or give body, color, or fragrance to the product. The basic functions of some of the more common ingredients found in creams and lotions are defined below.

Emollients are chemicals used to soften and smooth your skin. *Humectants* are substances that absorb and hold on to moisture and act as lubricants for your skin. In moisturizing creams and lotions, emollients and humectants are the major active ingredients. These are the ingredients that work on your behalf, not on behalf of the product. By this I mean that you might tend to think that nearly all the ingredients in a particular product serve some skin moisturizing functions. You will see shortly, however, that the majority of the ingredients in a moisturizing lotion, other than the emollients and humectants, actually have little to do with moisturizing your skin. In other words, a lot of what goes into cosmetics does nothing for your skin, but is needed to manufacture and preserve the product.

The following ingredients commonly found in many cosmetics are needed in order to satisfactorily blend the various ingredients and to keep the product stable:

Solvents are the carrier liquids into which other chemical ingredients are dissolved. Water, for example, is the solvent for all the chemicals in our blood. *Emulsifying agents (surfactants)* are used for their surface-acting properties to mix oil and water in order to make creams and lotions. As you know, oil and water ordinarily cannot be mixed together. Emulsifying agents are frequently referred to by a variety of other names, such as detergents, foaming agents, etc. (see Table 1), when they are expressly incorporated into a particular product for those purposes. When emulsifiers are included in a product for their detergent properties, you can consider them to be working for you. When they are included for their other properties, such as foaming, they are really working primarily for the product, not you. *Emulsion stabilizers* keep oil and water mixed and prevent their separating out. *Preservatives* prevent spoilage by germs and make refrigeration unnecessary; *antioxidants* prevent the fats and oils in cosmetics from becoming rancid by preventing their reaction with oxygen in the air; and *chemical stabilizers* extend shelf-life by slowing down other chemical changes. *Viscosity builders* add to the thickness of oil and water suspensions to create a heavy, "cushiony" feel, while *thickening, stiffening, and suspending agents* are chemicals used to solidify (thicken) a product. *Gellants* are particular kinds of thickeners that, when combined with alcohol, acetone, or water, make transparent gels that liquefy (thin) when you apply them to your skin.

Finally, to the basic chemical ingredients listed in Table 1, manufacturers may add specific colors (e.g., D&C, FD&C colors, iron oxides, bismuth oxychlorides, etc.), powders, detergents, sunscreens, conditioners, fragrances, or exotic additives (e.g., herbals, aloe, allantoin, etc.) needed to make the particular finished product. Added ingredients are placed there largely to work for you or to attract you—to give you the right shade of cosmetic you need, a pleasing fragrance, or a soft feel, etc. As a simple example, to make a creamy foundation makeup, a manufacturer will blend specific pigments and fragrances into their basic formula for a cream base.

By now it should be apparent that seeing a long list of ingredients with impressive chemical names on a cosmetic label does not necessarily make that product any better than its competitors. Furthermore, most of the ingredients included in these products by the manufacturer, despite their imposing scientific or exotic names, are not really there as active ingredients for your benefit. As I said in Chapter 1, exotic ingredients generally do nothing for a cosmetic except make it more expensive.

Prove this to yourself the next time you are at the cosmetics counter. Compare two or three products such as undermakeup moisturizers or foundation makeups that have the same function but differ greatly in price. You will probably see many of the same ingredients listed first in both the expensive and less expensive products. In the more expensive product, you will probably find an exotic ingredient listed someplace toward the end of the ingredient list, such as collagen, aloe vera, or algae. Very often it is the exotic ingredient that is being advertised as the magical property to make your skin younger or healthier, while, in fact, it is the first few ingredients on the list as the *emollients* that are important for you. The addition of exotic ingredients (and the fancier packaging) are largely responsible for the higher prices. With Table 1 in mind, and a healthy skepticism about any advertising claims that sound too good to be true, you will be able to make better choices for less money. I'm not saying that it's not okay to buy more expensive cosmetics when you like the look or feel of them. It's fine as long as you recognize the reasons you are buying them—and are not misled into believing that you're getting so much more for your money.

HYPOALLERGENIC AND
OTHER CATCHY TERMS

Overall, allergic reactions to cosmetics are relatively rare and usually have to do with an individual's own unique response to specific ingredients. When applied to cosmetics, the term *hypo-allergenic* may give you the impression that these cosmetics are either nonallergenic or much less allergenic than other cosmetics not so labeled. This is not necessarily the case, however.

About forty years ago, a few manufacturers began to produce cosmetics from which some ingredients considered at the time to be more commonly allergenic, such as certain fragrances, were eliminated. These cosmetics were referred to as hypoallergenic. In addition, these manufacturers made their product ingredient lists readily available to physicians who requested them. Since that time, many major manufacturers have realized that it makes good business sense to eliminate potential sensitizers from their products. Therefore, to my patients who ask about the advantages of using hypoallergenic cosmetics, I generally respond: What manufacturer in its right mind is going to produce products that are potentially highly allergenic to many people? In fact, most major brands today are basically hypoallergenic, whether or not it is stated on the product packaging.

Finally, being hypoallergenic does not mean, as many people mistakenly assume, that a cosmetic cannot cause an allergic reaction. After all, the basic oils, waxes, alcohol, and perfumes in these cosmetics are identical to those contained in most other cosmetics. Hypoallergenic does mean, however, that the manufacturer has made an effort to eliminate as many of the known sensitizers from their products as they could. Unfortunately, no company has yet been able to make a completely nonallergenic cosmetic.

Manufacturers may use other phrases to describe their cosmetics, phrases intended to assure you of the safety and lack of allergenicity of their products. Terms such as *natural, organic,* and *herbal* are often used interchangeably. To reiterate my remarks in Chapter 1 about soaps bearing these same labels, the fruit, vegetable, and herbal extracts contained are often so heavily processed to prevent them from becoming rancid they lose any natural benefits they might have had. Again, there is no scientific evidence to show that their inclusion in any product serves any useful function at all.

Phrases such as *doctor-tested, dermatologist-tested,* or *allergy-tested* are also frequently used in product advertising. These claims are meant to lure you into a sense of security, but what they *don't* tell you is *who* did the testing, *how* they did the tests, and *how many* tests were really performed. Without this kind of information, you really have little guarantee of product value, and much cause for skepticism.

COSMETIC ALLERGIES

Allergies to cosmetics may cause itching, redness, swelling, and blistering. While it commonly results from the use of a newly purchased cosmetic, a cosmetic allergy can develop after months or even years of use of the same product. In general, people with personal or strong family histories of asthma, hay fever, hives, or dust and dander allergies appear to be somewhat more likely to demonstrate sensitivities to certain cosmetics, particularly those that contain perfumes.

If you should become allergic to a specific brand of cosmetic, don't despair. You don't necessarily have to give up using all brands of that type of product. With a little experimentation, you may be able to find the specific culprit, eliminate it, and still continue using cosmetics.

For the sake of illustration, let's say that you developed an allergy to a particular brand of reddish cream blush. The first thing you should do, of course, is to discontinue the use of that particular blush. Allow the allergy to clear completely, which may take up to two weeks. Then choose another brand of red cream blush. If, after three straight days of use, you don't develop allergic symptoms to the new product, it is not likely that your allergy is to the red pigment, but to some other ingredient in the original product, probably the fragrance. At this point, you can continue to use the new product.

If you do develop the same allergy with the new red cream blush, it is possible that you are allergic to the red color. Let the allergy clear, then switch to a different color cream blush and try it for three straight days. If you have no further problems, you may continue to use this blush.

If, however, the different color cream blush produces an allergic reaction, you are most likely allergic to one of the standard ingredients comprising the base of most brands of blushes. At this point, you have two choices: Resign yourself to giving up blushes altogether, or consult a dermatologist about having patch testing performed to find out exactly which ingredient(s) caused your problem (Chapter 15).

UNDERMAKEUP COLOR
TONERS AND
MASKING COSMETICS

Until now I have discussed the use of cosmetics for the purpose of beautifying otherwise normal skin. However, there exist a number of skin conditions, some present at birth, others acquired later in life, for which cosmetics are needed as camouflage. For some of these skin conditions, the proper use of conventional cosmetics is all that is necessary to conceal them. However, certain more severely disfiguring skin conditions require special cosmetics and techniques for application and removal. For some people, camouflage cosmetics have made it possible for them to go out and face the world with greater confidence. Yet because the number of people who need them is rather small, masking cosmetics are not heavily advertised, and many consumers are not even aware that they are available.

Undermakeup color toners, which come in lotion, gel, cream, or stick forms, can be used to change the color of your complexion or to even out blotchy skin discolorations. As the name suggests, an undermakeup toner is intended to be applied as a thin film to your face *under* your ordinary makeup. If, for example, you have a very ruddy complexion or have a dense network of tiny "broken" blood vessels on your face and nose (the so-called "drinker's nose"), you can use a green shaded undermakeup toner to reduce the flushed appearance. On the other hand, if you have a sallow complexion, you should choose either a red or a reddish-brown undermakeup toner in order to brighten your complexion. If you have these kinds of skin color problems, I also suggest that you seek the advice of a professional cosmetician to help you choose the right shade of toner for your specific problem and to show you how best to apply it.

When scars or other disfiguring marks, completely depigmented spots (*vitiligo*), deep discolorations of the face, ears, and neck (such as large age spots and large port wine stains) need to be masked, special camouflage cosmetics can be helpful. They can completely conceal many types of skin problems, but work best on flatter discolorations. On the down side, masking cosmetics tend to be quite expensive. Owing to their thickness, they also tend to aggravate acne in some people who are acne prone. COVERMARK and DERMABLEND are the two major brands of masking cosmetics I recommend.

Masking makeups, which are opaque, sunproof, and waterproof, are applied in a different manner from ordinary foundation makeups. They must be patted gently onto your skin and then set with a setting powder. Afterward, you can apply your regular makeup directly over the camouflage cosmetic. Once the masking makeup is dried and set, you may go ocean or pool swimming without fear of its coming off. At the end of the day, the camouflage is removed with a cleansing cream.

SKIN DYES

Vitiligo is a distressing condition in which patches of otherwise normal skin completely lose their color. In darker-complected people, the contrast between the white vitiligo spots and the surrounding normal skin can be striking and disfiguring. VITA-

DYE and DY-O-DERM, two nonprescription skin dyes, can occasionally be effectively used to conceal vitiligo. These products contain a nontoxic skin dye, dihydroxyacetone, that stains the uppermost layer of the skin. A small amount of the brownish-colored liquid is placed on the vitiligo area and allowed to dry. More is added until the color of the vitiligo spots more closely matches that of the surrounding normally pigmented skin. While they are water-fast, skin dyes must be reapplied every three to four days, since some of the stain is continuously lost as the upper layer of dead skin cells is shed. When an individual is fortunate enough to achieve a good color match, this type of therapy is practical, reasonably convenient, and inexpensive. When a good match cannot be obtained, masking cosmetics can be helpful. In any case, consultation with a dermatologist for vitiligo is advisable.

5

*Caring for Your
Hair and Scalp*

A healthy head of hair is a vital part of your appearance. Much money is spent on products that are supposed to make hair glow, and look "alive." There are products to clean and condition your hair, "feed," "nourish," bleach, dye, straighten, and curl it. And then there are products to restore your hair after you have finished doing all those other things to it. With such a wide selection, choosing the right products can be difficult. Moreover, if you have a scalp problem, such as itching or dandruff, the right choice of hair care products is especially important. However, some basic information about your hair, and scalp and hair care products, can lead you to make the appropriate choices.

Despite what you hear about "nourishing" your hair to make it look "alive," your hair is a nonliving, protein fiber. Every strand of your hair grows from hair roots that are located deep within the follicles (pores) of your scalp, and your scalp is the home, so to speak, of the living hair roots. Hair strands themselves are composed of a dead fibrous protein called *keratin.* A typical hair shaft contains an inner portion, called the *cortex,* and a "fish-scale-like" outer portion called the *cuticle* (Figure 2). As the diagram shows, the cuticle is normally arranged in overlapping layers and serves to protect the cortex from fraying and splitting. For all intents and purposes, hair fibers are analo-

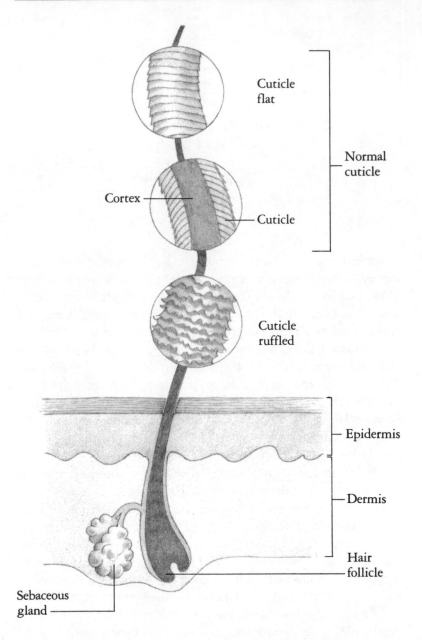

FIGURE 2. Hair follicle and hair shaft

gous to clothing fibers; they were never alive and cannot be brought to life.

The number of hair follicles that you have, and their arrangement on your scalp, are inherited. The color, texture, type, and length of your hair are also family traits. Normally, the number of scalp hairs in a full head of hair ranges from eighty thousand to one hundred twenty thousand. Blondes tend to have more, but finer hairs, brunettes fewer, but coarser hairs, and redheads the fewest, but coarsest hairs.

An average person with a normal head of hair loses between fifty and one hundred hairs per day. Under normal circumstances, lost hairs are replaced by an equal number of new hairs, which are made in the hair root within the follicle below the scalp surface. Your hair, which grows faster during the summer than in the winter, grows about a half an inch per month. Growth occurs in cycles—a growing phase, a resting phase, and a falling out phase. In general, hair grows for approximately one to two years before falling out and being replaced. Since most of your hairs are in a growing phase at any time, you often are not aware of your average daily hair loss.

SHAMPOOS

The most important ingredient in any shampoo is the cleansing agent, known as the detergent. The main job of any shampoo is to remove dirt and excess oil. As you learned in Chapter 1, regular toilet soap is one form of detergent. Fifty years ago hair cleansing was done routinely with body soaps. Today we use synthetic detergent shampoos. Hard water, which contains relatively high amounts of calcium, reduces the cleansing power of regular soap and forms a scum deposit. The main advantage of the often expensive synthetic detergent shampoos is that, unlike basic toilet soap, they may be used with hard water without leaving a scum residue on your hair, which in turn can leave your hair dull, lusterless, and difficult to comb or manage. But for this property, however, synthetic detergents are really no better hair cleansers than regular soap. Besides, scum deposits can be rather easily rinsed off your hair with acidic substances such as lemon juice, vinegar, and beer. In fact, it was probably from their original use—rinsing hard water soap scum from hair—that lemon juice and beer earned their reputation as being especially good for hair. Other than their mild acidity, they have no special properties.

Synthetic detergents are sometimes referred to as *surfactants*—chemicals that have the ability to grab hold of oils and greases, at the same time attracting water to rinse them away. Cosmetic chemists have created literally dozens of surfactant detergents, which are usually classified in four basic groups: *anionic, cationic, amphoteric*, and *nonionic* detergents. Shampoos generally contain more than one detergent. Those intended for normal and oily hair are formulated by increasing the amount of strengths of the detergents. Shampoos for dry hair contain conditioners, compounds that restore some of the oils that the detergents in the shampoos wash away, in order to remoisturize the hair.

Shampoos for adults usually contain anionic detergents. The milder "no-tears" shampoos for children contain amphoteric detergents but do not contain added ingredients, such as perfumes, which can sting the eyes. Cationic and nonionic detergents are stronger cleansers, but have been associated with eye irritations, and so are generally no longer included in most shampoos.

Manufacturers have formulated shampoos as creams, lotions, gels, and pastes. In addition to the detergents, shampoos contain fragrances, colorings, thickening agents, and foaming and lathering agents. (Contrary to what you may think, a shampoo need *not* lather well in order to be effective.) These additives affect the look, feel, and smell of the various brands of shampoos, and frequently determine your personal preference for one preparation over another.

Some shampoos are touted as being "pH-balanced" or "acid-balanced." Detergents, which are usually alkaline, tend to ruffle the cuticles of your hair (the outer coatings of the hair shaft). When this happens, your hair can appear dull, lifeless, and be difficult to manage. This ruffling effect on your cuticles usually disappears on its own within a day or two as your natural hair oils reaccumulate. However, to speed the process, most companies acidify their shampoos by including citric or tartaric acids. In advertising jargon this is called pH-balancing.

In summary, a shampoo is basically a cleansing cosmetic for your hair and is quite similar to a mild dishwashing liquid. In fact, if you wish, you could safely use a mild commercial dishwashing liquid for shampooing your hair and save a fortune.

MEDICATED SHAMPOOS

Medicated shampoos contain ingredients intended to correct or prevent particular scalp problems, such as itching, dandruff, or scalp dermatitis (seborrheic dermatitis). *No shampoo can either restore or treat thinning hair.* Because they are meant to treat specific conditions, they are classified as drugs and are under Food and Drug Administration regulation. Unlike cosmetics, the safety of medicated shampoos must be tested to FDA satisfaction.

A variety of substances that are available in nonprescription medicated shampoos have been found helpful in controlling itching scalp, dandruff, flakiness, and even the more troublesome conditions of seborrheic dermatitis and scalp psoriasis. Through the years zinc pyrithione, sulfur, salicylic acid, selenium sulfide, and tar derivatives have been found particularly effective.

The medications contained in these shampoos have a variety of different functions. Zinc pyrithione and sulfur are used for their antiseptic abilities, sulfur and salicylic acid for their keratolytic (peeling, descaling) effects, and selenium sulfide and tars for their ability to slow down epidermal growth rate. For mild cases of itching scalp and dandruff, I usually advise patients to start with shampoos containing zinc pyrithione, such as HEAD AND SHOULDERS shampoo, ZINCON shampoo, or DANEX shampoo, and using them at least three times a week. For more troublesome or persistent problems, I suggest SELSUN-BLUE (selenium), SEBULEX (sulfur/salicylic acids) shampoo, IONIL PLUS (salicylic acid) shampoo, or T-GEL (tar) shampoo. You can use these shampoos daily, if necessary, to achieve or maintain control of your problem. Once this is accomplished, you may find that you need to use a medicated shampoo only once or twice a week to maintain control. To be effective, any medicated shampoo must be massaged well into your scalp and left on for at least five minutes in order to allow the active ingredients sufficient time to work.

Medicated shampoos can often leave your hair dry, lusterless, and smelling like medicine, even when they contain ingredients to specifically mitigate these effects. If you don't like the way your hair looks, feels, or smells after using a medicated shampoo, you can use your favorite conditioner as a final rinse. Tar shampoos tend to yellow gray hair and can occasionally cause an itchy, pimple-like inflammation (*folliculitis*) of your scalp when used too frequently. Less frequent use of the tar shampoos, or alternating them with other kinds of medicated or regular shampoos, will usually eliminate the problem.

CONDITIONING SHAMPOOS AND CONDITIONERS

Conditioners are ingredients specifically formulated to help restore your hair. A conditioning shampoo is a detergent shampoo to which conditioners have been added. On the other hand, the word conditioner has come to mean a product distinct from a shampoo and one created exclusively to restore your hair. A conditioner is intended to be used as an additional rinse *after* regular shampooing. In general, although a one-product-does-

it-all would be ideal, the basic functions of detergents and conditioners run counter to each other. For that reason, your hair
will usually benefit more from rinsing with a separate conditioner after shampooing, rather than using a conditioning
shampoo. However, for some of you with less problematic hair,
a conditioning shampoo may prove not only convenient, but
quite satisfactory.

In general, conditioners are especially useful for hair damaged by bleaching, dyeing, permanent-waving, excessive sun
exposure, and chlorine pool swimming. There are basically three
types of hair conditioning products. One type contains oils, such
as lanolin derivatives, balsam, and vegetable oils, which are
meant to replace the oils that your detergent shampoo has
washed away. A second type, called protein conditioners because they contain proteins—frequently "hydrolyzed animal
proteins"—binds to your hair to make it feel softer and look
shinier and fuller. The proteins in this type of conditioner can
also *temporarily* bind split ends and smooth roughened hairs.
Quarternary ammonium compounds constitute a third type of
conditioning agent. These compounds are used to prevent "flyaway" hair and make hair more manageable by reducing static
electricity.

Herbal additives, egg, and lemon juice add little to the
benefit of the conditioners and much to their price. And the so-
called "self-adjusting" conditioners, which are supposed to do
more for hair that needs it and less for hair that doesn't, offer
no particular advantages. As a rule, your hair will take just
what it needs and not more from any brand of conditioner. As
with all cosmetics, in the final analysis your ultimate choice of
conditioner remains a matter of personal preference. If your hair
looks limp or slightly greasy after using a conditioner, you probably didn't need one in the first place.

No chapter on general hair care would be complete without
some general do's and don'ts. Do shampoo your hair as often as
you need to control oiliness and flaking. For those of you with
dry hair, shampooing once a week may be all that you require.

However, if you need to wash your hair more frequently, you will be happy to learn that *daily shampooing will neither damage your hair nor cause hair loss*. Do pat-dry your hair gently after shampooing. Don't vigorously towel dry your hair and don't brush it while it is still wet. Instead, comb it with a wide-toothed comb, let it dry, and then brush gently if you need to.

Brushing your hair gently every day can supplement shampooing by removing scales, dirt, and tangles while adding luster to your hair. Don't brush excessively and don't brush your scalp. Scalp brushing does not increase circulation; it only irritates your scalp. I recommend that you use only natural bristle brushes. Natural bristles are usually made from boar's hairs, which are tapered at the ends and are less likely to scratch your scalp. Synthetic bristles, generally made of nylon, are usually untapered and blunt tipped; hence, they are most likely to scratch.

Blow-drying need not be damaging to your hair. If you keep the blow-dryer at least six to twelve inches from your scalp, you should be able to prevent burning or overdrying your hair or scalp. Adjust your blow-dryer to a slow air-flow and cooler settings. These settings will still allow you to style your hair properly, but will be less damaging. It is also important that you not attempt to keep blow-drying your hair until it is completely dry; instead, you should try to leave your hair slightly damp.

Finally, avoid tight hairstyles or hairstyling methods that place a great deal of tension on your hair or scalp. The prolonged practice of tight plaiting and the use of brush rollers have been associated with a form of occasionally temporary, yet often permanent, hair loss called *traction alopecia*. The hair roots can sustain permanent damage where hairs have been pulled most tightly, and prolonged tension on the hairs themselves can result in hair breakage.

6

Changing Your Hair

All natural hair shades are actually variations of brown. This simply means that drab shades are brown with an excess of blue highlights, golden shades are brown with an excess of yellow color, and warm shades are brown with an excess of reddish color. Formulas and recipes for changing natural hair color have been used for thousands of years. These recipes usually contained plant extracts or metallic dyes, two of which are still being used. Today, over thirty-three million women and countless men spend over four hundred million dollars annually for hair coloring preparations.

Three basic groups of hair coloring products are currently available. They differ primarily on how long the new color they give will last. *Temporary* dyes give a color that is removable in one shampooing. *Semipermanent* dyes give your hair color that will last through about five to six shampoos. *Permanent* colorants last until your hair grows out. The majority of hair dyes used today employ aniline dyes, particularly paraphenylenediamine, a petroleum derivative.

Temporary (Acid) Dyes

Temporary dyes, which are also known as *rinses*, do not penetrate your hair, but instead coat it with water soluble colors (food colors). No permanent chemical reaction takes place, which is the reason that the color coating is usually removed with the next regular shampooing. Unfortunately, temporary hair colors can rub off on your pillowcase or clothes and can be bleached out to some extent by heavy perspiration. Temporary rinses, besides being easy and relatively safe to use, serve best to brighten and add highlights to your hair, even out streaked hair, and tone down gray or yellowed hair. Mild organic acids found in these rinses help to promote the binding of the dye to your hair. The acid dyes used in temporary preparations are frequently certified by the FDA, which means that the synthetic colors being used are highly purified, have been tested for safety, and generally do not require a patch test before use.

Semipermanent Hair Colors

Semipermanent colorants are able to last through between five and six shampooings. These preparations can add color to your hair, but cannot be used to make your hair lighter. They are excellent for coloring gray hair, to highlight blond hair, or to retouch hair between uses of permanent hair colorants. Since semipermanent rinses are simply shampooed in and require no developers, accelerators, or ammonia, they are convenient to use and relatively nondamaging to your hair and scalp. They happen to be a popular choice for men. Although allergies to semipermanent hair coloring preparations are rare, to be safe, you should follow the package directions and perform a patch test before using them. Directions for performing the test are usually included with the product instructions.

Permanent Hair Colorant (Tints)

Used more frequently than any other type of hair coloring preparations, permanent hair dyes (*oxidation dyes, tints*) are produced for home and professional salon use. The large selection of natural shades and the permanence of the tinting are the distinct advantages of these products. Unlike the other types of hair coloring agents, oxidation dyes can produce colors several shades lighter than your natural color. (For more drastic lightening, bleaching, which will be covered in the next section, is required.)

Permanent hair dyes are called oxidation dyes because in addition to the dye, a developer or oxidizing substance (usually 6 percent hydrogen peroxide) is needed to chemically react with the dye to produce the desired shade. The dye and developer are mixed right before use; after application they chemically react within the shafts of your hairs. Other ingredients are added to help the coloring agents penetrate into the hair shaft so that permanent coloration can take place.

Professional salons tend to use creme tint products, which are applied with a brush, swab, or applicator by the method called *parting and sectioning.* Most of the products intended primarily for home use are "shampoo-in" tints. "Shampoo-in" tints are easier to use, but generally do not cover gray as well.

Although infrequent, allergy to oxidation dyes does occur and you should perform a patch test as directed by the product manufacturer *before each use* to determine whether you have developed an allergy to the dye. Since allergic sensitivity to a dye may develop at any time, performing only one patch test when you first use a particular product is, therefore, not sufficient. Too frequent use of permanent colorants can weaken or damage your hair. In general, you should not use permanent hair colorants more than once every six to eight weeks.

BLEACHING AGENTS AND TONERS ("DOUBLE PROCESS")

If you want to drastically lighten the color of your hair, permanent dyes are usually not sufficient. Instead you will need to first bleach (strip) your hair, then color it. This two-step procedure is commonly referred to as the "double process." With ordinary (permanent) oxidation tints, the hydrogen peroxide in the developer serves as a bleaching agent. However, when you wish more dramatic lightening such as changing black or dark brown hair to flaxen blond, the amount of bleaching in a permanent tint would be inadequate. In this case a separate bleaching step is required to "strip" your hair of its natural color. Bleaching agents contain 6 percent hydrogen peroxide and an "accelerator" substance, usually a *persulfate*, to boost the bleaching reaction. They frequently contain ammonia, which is needed to ensure adequate bleaching.

After bleaching, a toner dye is used to achieve the right shade. The bleaching makes your hair reddish and strawlike; toners provide the finishing touch. Toners may either be semipermanent or permanent dye products. Frosting, tipping, streaking, or painting are merely variations of the double process in which only portions of your hair, rather than all of it, are bleached and toned.

Bleaching damages hair. Unfortunately, the peroxide bleaching step, which is essential, is in fact an attack on the hair proteins and causes your hair to be dry, brittle, and strawlike. As a result, bleached hair is more fragile than natural hair and requires after-shampoo conditioners to give it body and manageability. To minimize further damage, bleached hair should be manipulated very carefully and as little as possible; this means brushing, combing, or blow-drying very gently. In general, don't retint your hair more than once every four to six weeks, since this can result in further hair damage. Above all, carefully consider making any drastic changes in your hair color; the more drastic the change, the more damage is likely to be done. Finally, permanent-waving should be performed with caution on bleached hair. If you bleach your hair and also wish to have it permanently waved, I suggest you have it done by an experienced salon professional.

HENNA AND
METALLIC DYES

Two other nonoxidation—albeit permanent—dyes deserve mention: henna and metallic dyes. Henna, in use for thousands of years, is a plant extract. Part of its appeal rests on its being a safe, natural substance. Ground leaves and stems are applied to your scalp in the form of a pack, which is actually a paste made with hot water. The pack is left in place until the desired color is attained. However, the only color that can be obtained with pure henna is orange-red. To achieve any other colors, henna must be combined with petroleum-derivative dyes. When combined with other dyes, however, any advantages to using a product containing henna are lost.

Metallic dyes, which usually contain lead acetate, are also called "progressive" dyes. They require daily application to achieve progressive darkening of your hair. The lead reacts with the sulfur in your hair to produce the color. These products have enjoyed particular popularity among men who prefer to comb their color in. Metallic dyes usually result in intense, somewhat artificial colors. Furthermore, hair treated in this way can be difficult to permanently wave.

SETTING HAIR AND
ELECTRIC ROLLERS

Demand for curly or wavy hair swings with the fashion pendulum. Rearranging naturally straight or wavy hair to be more wavy or curly became very popular about twenty years ago and shows no sign of abating.

The specific shape of your hairs (i.e., whether they are curly, wavy, straight, etc.) is determined by two types of linkages of the protein molecules in them: strong sulfur bonds and weaker hydogen bonds. In general, temporary setting procedures, such as the simple use of water to style your hair, hairsetting preparations, and even electric rollers depend largely upon affecting the weaker hydrogen bonds. These bonds are first disrupted and then realigned to make the desired straight or curly hair. Longer lasting changes achieved with permanent-waving preparations work by breaking and rearranging the stronger sulfur bonds.

Setting lotions, which generally contain some kind of gum or resin, are applied after your hair has been shampooed and placed in rollers. These ingredients coat your hair and lock out moisture in order to keep the set longer.

For quick sets, electric rollers can give you a fairly good, if temporary set. The heat in electric rollers breaks the weaker hydrogen bonds in your hair. Hot-mist (steam-heated) rollers are generally better than straight electric rollers because the mist restores some of the moisture to the hair that plain heat normally takes away. Too frequent use of electric rollers, however, can leave your hair dry and brittle, particularly if you have tinted or bleached hair.

Home use of electric curling irons, while safe, may cause problems. In general, curling irons are hotter than electric curlers. If the heat is too low to break the protein bonds in your hair, curling will be unsatisfactory. On the other hand, if the heat generated is too high, your hair may become excessively dry, brittle, or even burned. I usually do not recommend curling irons for these reasons.

PERMANENT-WAVING

Permanent-waving and *hair straightening* are two other ways to give to your hair something that nature didn't. Permanent-waving, or cold-waving, as it is also known (since heat is no longer required), is a process for making straight hair wavy or curly. Hair straightening, as its name indicates, is a technique for doing just the reverse, i.e., making naturally curly or wooly hair straight. The object of the chemical reactions in these two processes is basically the same: to break the stronger linkages between the protein molecules in your hair and re-form them at new angles to give the desired effect.

For permanent-waving, the hair is usually wrapped around a small roller and then an alkaline waving solution or foam containing *ammonium thioglycollate* is applied. These steps break the protein bonds in your hair. The alkalinity of the solution permits deeper penetration of the bond-breaking chemical into your hairs. Depending upon the strength of the waving solution, the type of hair being permanented, and the type of wave desired, the waving solution may be left in place for between five and thirty minutes. In general, the weaker the waving solution and the larger the roller used, the larger and softer the waves will be. Next, an acidic solution containing hydrogen peroxide, the *neutralizer*, is applied to the hair. After several minutes, the rollers are removed, the hair is shampooed and then set.

As a rule it is more difficult to permanently wave fine, limp, brittle, wiry, or previously damaged hair. For short hair, permanents need to be repeated about once every three months; for longer hair, about once every six months.

HAIR STRAIGHTENING

There are three different types of chemical hair straighteners: thioglycollates, sodium hydroxide, and bisulfite straighteners. All of them act by breaking the chemical bonds in curly hair, permitting them to be rearranged.

Thioglycollates are the same chemicals found in permanent-waving lotions. For hair straightening, however, they are used in stronger concentrations. Straighteners are sold in cream and lotion forms. When thioglycollate solutions are used for hair straightening, they are referred to as *relaxing lotions*. These are applied to the hair and allowed to work for about twenty minutes, during which time the hair should be combed continually so that it will hang straight. Then a neutralizer is added. Combing should continue until the hair is fixed into its new straight shape. Finally, the hair is shampooed, set on giant rollers, and dried. Unfortunately, thioglycollate straighteners frequently do not give the desired degree of straightening.

Given their potential hazards, sodium hydroxide (alkali) straighteners are limited to salon usage. Sodium hydroxide, a very potent alkali, works on the hair rapidly—usually within five to ten minutes—to break the natural protein bonds. The hair then quickly relaxes with combing. A thorough rinsing of the hair neutralizes the chemical. However, the potential for severe scalp and skin irritation and burns exists, so precautions, such as protecting the skin near the scalp with a thick cream, should be taken. *Extreme care must also be taken to protect the eyes, since blindness could result.*

Bisulfite straighteners, sometimes referred to as "curl relaxers," are the most widely used home straightening agents. The bisulfite is applied to a damp scalp and then covered by a plastic cap for about fifteen minutes. This breaks chemical bonds in the hair. Next, the hair is rinsed and covered with an alkaline stabilizer. Bisulfite straighteners are generally mild on your hair and scalp, and effective.

The use of pomades, hot combing or ironing the hair for hair straightening have all been associated with problems and should be avoided. While oily or vaseline-like pomades are safe enough and serve merely to "plaster" down your hair and hold it in place, their thickness can clog your pores and lead to "pimples" (folliculitis) on the scalp. In addition, if you are predisposed toward acne, it, too, can flare up around the hairline and forehead. And certain of the ingredients in pomades can cause allergic reactions.

Hot combing or hot pressing has been associated with severe burns of the skin and scalp, damage to the hair itself, and patchy hair loss. The procedure consists of applying an oil to the hair after shampooing. Next, a heated metal pressing comb is run through the hair to straighten it. The high heat temporarily breaks the hair bonds. The straightening effect, however, is much reduced by exposure to environmental humidity or even sweat, and the hair soon returns to its normal curliness. I feel that the benefits of hot combing are not worth any of its risks.

Finally, the practice of using a steam iron to straighten the hair is one to be avoided. The risk of heat damage to the hair and accidental burning of the hair and scalp make this a particularly unwise procedure. Chemical straighteners, when used properly, make far more practical alternatives.

7

*Fighting Oily Skin
and Acne Blemishes*

In my experience, few other dermatologic conditions are surrounded by more myths and misconceptions than acne. Variously
called "teenage acne," "zits," pimples, or more technically, *acne
vulgaris*, acne is one of the most common problems seen in a
dermatologist's practice. While not life-threatening, it has long
been the cause of considerable emotional and physical suffering
for millions of people. The scarring that may result from uncontrolled, severe acne can adversely affect the quality of a person's life well after its active stages have disappeared. Acne is
nothing to joke about. The embarrassment and loss of self-
esteem caused by acne and acne scarring can be serious problems. Fortunately, for most people, acne frequently is only a
relatively mild condition that can be rather easily controlled
by proper facial hygiene and the use of the right over-the-
counter preparations.

FACTS AND FANCIES
ABOUT ACNE

The exact cause of acne is not known, but a tendency to develop
it seems to run in certain families, i.e., the predisposition for

the development of acne appears to be inherited. It has been estimated that about 80 percent of adolescents develop acne to some extent. Acne vulgaris is not an infectious disease caused by bacteria, as some people think, but a kind of *inflammation* of the skin.

Figure 3 summarizes the usual stages in acne formation. Normally, the lining of your hair follicles sheds its surface layer of dead cells every day. These shed cells are then "washed" to the surface of your skin by secretions of your oil glands. If you are predisposed to acne, your shed lining cells exhibit a kind of increased stickiness. They tend to stick together, form a plug, and clog the openings of your pores. When a plug sits exposed in the pore opening directly at the surface of the skin, it is called an open *comedo* (plural: comedones) or *blackhead* (Figure

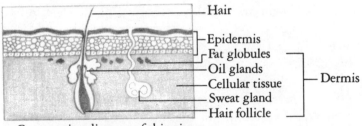

a. Cross section diagram of skin tissue

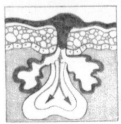

b. Blackhead

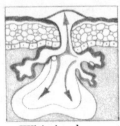

c. Whitehead

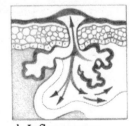

d. Inflammatory lesions— pimples, pustules, cysts

FIGURE 3. Steps in acne formation

3b), owing to the fact that the exposed surface of the plug is black in color. When the plug lies below the surface and is not open to the surface, it is called a closed comedo or *whitehead* (Figure 3c).

Dead cells and oil gland secretion continue to accumulate within clogged pores. Skin bacteria, called *proprionobacterium acnes*, that are present within your hair follicles begin to work on the accumulated materials within clogged pores and break them down into very irritating substances called *fatty acids*. Whiteheads, if exposed to excessive mechanical pressure from without, or excessive irritation from the fatty acids within them, may rupture or begin leaking the irritating fatty acids into the surrounding skin below the surface. Your body responds by initiating inflammation, resulting in the familiar pimples, pustules, and abscesses typical of acne (Figure 3d).

Other than being cosmetically distressing, blackheads, unlike whiteheads, generally do not lead to further problems. The black substance of the blackhead is *not* dirt, as is often thought, but is probably oxidized skin pigment. In fact, you might think of it as a kind of "skin-rust."

The misconception (about the supposed "dirt" in blackheads) may be responsible for the old myth about acne being a disease of dirty people. And that myth may have been responsible for the common belief that frequent facial cleansing was the best way of both treating and preventing acne. We now know that this is not true. In fact, scrubbing your face can even make matters worse. Superscrubbing can precipitate acne by rupturing whiteheads under your skin and releasing the irritating fatty acids. Secondly, superscrubbing can dry out and irritate your skin so much that you may find it too uncomfortable to tolerate the application of real anti-acne therapies to your face.

Androgens, male hormones found normally in men and in smaller amounts in women, are responsible for stimulating your oil glands to secrete. They have also been linked to the oil gland overactivity and oily complexions seen in many teenagers.

Changes in temperature, the amount of sun exposure you receive, and your emotions can affect how oily your skin is at any time. Your own skin surface oils play little role in the development of acne; the steps leading to acne formation, as you saw earlier, actually occur *below* the surface of the skin.

COMMON MISCONCEPTIONS ABOUT ACNE

Acne is surrounded by a number of other myths and misconceptions which also need to be dispelled. Chief among these is the one about acne being caused by certain foods. Although some people are so convinced of this that it becomes a real task to disabuse them of it, nevertheless *acne vulgaris is neither caused by nor made worse by eating the wrong foods*. There is no reason, at least as far as your acne is concerned, to avoid eating chocolates, fried foods, colas, nuts, potato chips, candy, ice cream, or pizza. (Of course, these foods are *not* particularly healthy for your heart or blood vessels.) I tell all my new patients with acne that since they are already miserable enough, there is no need to increase their misery by eliminating the foods they enjoy.

Foods high in iodine, however, such as shellfish, kelp, iodized table salts, and mineral supplements containing iodine may aggravate preexistent acne. You should reduce your intake of these foods or completely avoid them. The mineral iodine is usually included in most commercial multivitamins with mineral supplements. If you routinely require a multivitamin and mineral supplement, avoid the iodine by taking a plain multivitamin tablet and the individual supplement you specifically need.

Acne is brought on by sex is another popular myth, and one that often arouses a good deal of guilt and embarrassment in some adolescents. However, there is absolutely no medical substantiation for this belief. The only link between sex and acne is that, following puberty, the same increase in production of male hormones (androgens) that affects sexual behavior and development is also responsible for increasing oil gland secretion.

Another favorite misconception is that acne can be caused by having long hair or by letting your hair rest on your forehead. In fact, the surface oils coating your hairs play little role in acnegenesis.

Still another misconception is that acne is exclusively a teenage problem. Disappointment, frustration, and anger frequently follow when acne sufferers learn otherwise. For some people, the discovery that the stroke of midnight of their twentieth birthday does not miraculously bring an end to their "teenage" acne problem comes as a jolt. For a sizable number of acne sufferers, particularly women, the condition persists into their twenties, thirties, or even later. Some outgrow it only to have it recur later on. A patient of mine who had acne in her forties complained to me that she was convinced she was destined to go straight "from acne to wrinkles."

Finally, there's the myth that sunbathing is one of the best treatments for acne. The majority of people with acne do observe a temporary improvement in their condition following sun exposure. Moreover, a "healthy"-looking tan can mask acne blemishes. However, a large number of those who initially improve with sun exposure may notice a pronounced increase in whiteheads on their faces about a month later, which may immediately precede a new flare-up of their acne problem. The penetrating and damaging ultraviolet rays of the sun, which are able to reach below the skin surface, can make worse the basic, underlying pore-plugging problem. Furthermore, whenever you overexpose yourself to sunlight in hopes of temporarily improving your acne problem, you must balance this against the potential, irreversible, long-term damaging effects of the sun. The same holds true for using artificial ultraviolet light sources, such as sunlamps, for acne control.

AGGRAVATING FACTORS

Physical and emotional stresses aggravate acne. While nervous tension is *not* the cause of acne, there is no doubt in my mind that increased emotional stress plays an important aggravating role in acne. I frequently warn my patients that their acne is most likely to flare up at certain particularly stressful times: final exams, a heavy date, a fight with a lover or mate, involvement in divorce proceedings, getting married, a death in the family, and dealing with a miserable boss. Physical stresses on your body such as menstruation (most commonly during the week preceding your period), high humidity, hormonal abnormalities, undergoing major or even minor surgery, colds, or seasonal allergies have also been associated with acne flare-ups.

Acne may also result from using certain kinds of medications. Hormones, antiepileptic drugs, antituberculosis agents, lithium, and corticosteroids used either orally or topically may precipitate acne or may aggravate a preexistent acne condition. Interestingly, the use of birth control pills can clear acne in some women and make it worse in others. Pregnancy may also do this.

Exposure to certain agents in the workplace, such as industrial cutting oils, grease, and chemicals like PCB's can also precipitate acne. Even greasy cosmetics may contribute to it.

Lastly, after debunking so many acne myths and misconceptions, I must remind you that one old belief still obtains: *Keep your hands away from your face.* Any unnecessary manipulation of your face can lead to the rupturing of the whiteheads under your skin, resulting in a new breakout. For the same reason, you should avoid resting your chin on your hands and using tight headbands, headsets, or chinstraps.

WHAT YOU CAN DO
FOR YOURSELF

Before getting down to the specifics of self-treatment for acne, I would like to stress a few basic don'ts and a few important skin care rules. Don't superscrub your face! Don't use harsh soaps, abrasive soaps, highly alkaline soaps, deodorant soaps, or so-called "acne soaps." These soaps are generally much too drying. Furthermore, as I mentioned in Chapter 1, since soaps by nature are meant to be immediately rinsed off, any truly active ingredients contained in the soap do not have sufficient contact time with your skin to be of any significant value. Even if you have extremely oily skin, you will find that gentle cleansers coupled with anti-acne topicals are usually more than sufficient to keep oiliness suppressed. You are better off using superfatted soaps, transparent soaps, soapless soaps, and washable lotions. You need to keep your skin moist, supple, and in good enough condition to tolerate the application of specific anti-acne remedies. For choosing and using the right facial cleanser, follow the specific recommendations provided in Chapter 1.

Don't use abrasive sponges or washcloths for washing your face, and never superscrub! You don't want to leave your skin overly dry. It will do nothing for your acne or your appearance except to make your skin look flaky and dry. Again, you especially do *not* want to make yourself so dry that it will become too uncomfortable when you apply real acne medications.

Most topical anti-acne remedies have the unfortunate side effect of leaving your face a shade on the dry side. If you couple this with a misguided attempt to "dry" up your acne by excessive scrubbing, your face may become painfully dry. Many people do, in fact, show up at my office for their first visit after having tried on their own to scrub away and dry up their pimples. Despite all the scrubbing, they come in with a faceful of acne, but with skin so dry and flaky that they can barely open their mouths without discomfort. Instead of giving up scrubbing, some people add to their problems by applying heavy, oily, moisturizing lotions and cosmetics to counter the dryness for which they themselves are responsible. Such heavy preparations only aggravate the acne by further clogging the pores, not to mention increasing the frustration, defeat, and despair of the sufferer.

NONPRESCRIPTION ACNE MEDICATIONS

Four main ingredients are commonly found in most nonprescription anti-acne medications: sulfur, resorcinol, salicylic acid, and benzoyl peroxide. These active ingredients are used either alone or in combination in the various commercially available formulations. Most products for acne treatment are sold as creams, gels, or lotions.

Anti-acne products containing sulfur and sulfur combined with resorcinol have been used for generations. These ingredients are primarily *keratolytic* (peeling) and antibacterial agents. Their most important function, however, is not in preventing new pimples, but in dealing with those blemishes already present by speeding healing. Sulfur and resorcinol frequently come in flesh-tinted creams and lotions that can serve as a cover-up cosmetic. This particular function is usually more important for men who have reservations about using conventional cosmetic foundation makeups.

If you choose to use a flesh-tinted product, be sure to "feather" the edges of the preparation after you apply it in order to blend it better with the surrounding skin. On the down side, flesh-tinted topicals often do not precisely match your skin color. You also may occasionally find them difficult to completely wash off in the morning. Furthermore, they have a tendency to make dark skin look somewhat whitish and flaky. However, I advise patients to use REZAMID lotion and CLEARASIL'S ADULT CARE cream. Both are flesh-tinted.

VLEMASQUE, a sulfur-containing mask, deserves special note. This product, which is intended to be applied thickly to the skin, left on as a mask for twenty to thirty minutes, and completely rinsed off, is usually used for treating the pustules, abscesses, and acne cysts of moderately severe and severe inflammatory acne. Most patients not only find the mask soothing, but enjoy the fact that they do not need to keep a medication on their faces overnight.

Another traditional acne medication, salicylic acid, is usually reserved for mild cases of acne and those in which blackheads are a particular problem. Salicylic acid works primarily as a peeling agent to loosen and soften thick-clogged pores. Salicylic acid, like sulfur and resorcinol products, does little to prevent the formation of new acne blemishes. STRI-DEX MEDICATED PADS, which come in regular or maximum strengths, and SALIGEL are products I suggest to my patients. The alcohol bases of these preparations also help to remove oiliness, which can make you feel more comfortable and look cleaner and fresher. If you use STRI-DEX MEDICATED PADS, I suggest you start by using the regular strength. If no improvement is seen, but no irritation has occurred within two to three weeks, you should switch to the maximum-strength pads.

Benzoyl peroxide, an anti-acne medication which has come into wide usage in the past decade, is the only nonprescription medication that is capable of preventing new acne lesions. It does this in several ways: It penetrates your hair follicles and kills the acne bacteria, and also causes a mild peeling on the inside of the follicles and thereby helps to unplug your pores.

Benzoyl peroxide gels are generally felt to be more effective than benzoyl peroxide creams or lotions. Most benzoyl peroxide gels, however, require a doctor's prescription. CLEAR BY DESIGN (2.5 percent gel and FOSTEX BPO (5 percent and 10 percent) gel are gels available without prescription. I suggest beginning with the 2.5 percent gel, since the 5 percent or 10 percent gels do not seem to work any better, and tend to be considerably more drying and irritating to your skin. Be especially careful to avoid your eyelid and lip areas when applying benzoyl peroxides, as these areas may become extremely irritated.

NEUTROGENA'S ACNE MASK is a relatively new topical benzoyl peroxide preparation. Like VLEMASQUE, it is applied thickly to your skin to make a mask and then is washed off in twenty minutes. Dryness has not been a common complaint and once again, as with VLEMASQUE, most people enjoy the fact that they need not sleep with it on.

Unfortunately, most of the anti-acne topicals just described tend to leave your skin dry. Those with very oily complexions may like this; most people do not.

To minimize the drying and irritating effects of acne remedies, I recommend facial cleansing with a gentle soap or washable lotion not more than twice daily. The best time to apply acne medications is at bedtime, but no sooner than one-half hour after facewashing. The effects of almost any topical medication are enhanced by applying them to moist skin, but this applies as well to their side effects. The unwanted dryness caused by almost all acne medications will also be enhanced by applying them to moist skin. Therefore, you should wait until your skin is thoroughly dry before applying the medication. If after following all the right steps, you still find your skin too dry, you might try applying a moisturizer in the morning. CETAPHIL lotion or AQUACARE HP can serve as under-makeup moisturizers.

For moderately severe cases of acne, I frequently suggest the use of a combination of different acne medications applied nightly in a rotation. For example, one might use REZAMID lotion the first night, STRI-DEX MEDICATED PADS on the second night, and CLEAR BY DESIGN gel on the third. You should continue the rotation until you achieve satisfactory improvement, at which point you can reduce the number of times per week that you use each medication. A typical maintenance regimen would consist of using REZAMID lotion, for example, on Monday night, CLEAR BY DESIGN gel on Thursday night, and SALIGEL on Saturday night.

Women frequently ask me about which brands of cosmetics are least likely to aggravate their acne condition. Frankly, the brand is less important than the *type* you use. For acne conditions, do use the following: oil-free moisturizers, powder or gel blushers, and water-based foundations. If you must wear heavier, oilier cosmetics, be sure to remove them as soon as possible and follow that by applying your anti-acne therapy.

Embarrassing oiliness and shiny facial skin can be handled by simply blotting your skin with a soft facial tissue. If simple blotting is insufficient, you can periodically swab your face with alcohol towelettes (the kind your doctor uses to clean your skin before an injection). Each towelette comes individually wrapped and can be conveniently carried in your pocketbook. WITCH HAZEL lotion or SEBA-NIL (contains acetone) lotion are also astringents for control of greasiness. You should not use any of these products too frequently. Excessive use of astringents can overdry your skin and make matters worse.

When choosing any anti-acne remedies, remember that no one product is right for every person's skin. If you experience burning, itching, redness, or swelling following the use of any medication, you should immediately discontinue its use. *Caution*: moderately severe and severe acne are the types most likely to result in permanent scarring when proper treatment is delayed or when improperly treated. If you see no reasonable improvement in your acne condition after three or four weeks of self-treatment, you should consult a dermatologist.

8

*Dealing with Excess
Facial Hair*

Hirsutism, or *hypertrichosis,* refers to having excess hair anywhere on the body. On a woman's face, this generally translates into the coarsening of hair texture or the presence of heavy hair growth, usually on the upper lip, chin, and cheeks. Growth of excess facial hair can be psychologically distressing and even emotionally debilitating. The large majority of women with excess facial hair do not have any underlying medical conditions to account for it.

For many women, excess facial hair simply represents a familial or racial characteristic. Familial or racially associated excess facial hair is considered normal and part of normal growth and development. For example, persons of Mediterranean and Semitic origins are generally hairier and have darker hair than those of Scandinavian and North European extraction. Orientals, American Indians, and blacks are the least hairy. In addition, the appearance of excess facial hair in many women slightly before, or more frequently after, menopause is considered a normal developmental occurrence. The reasons for excess hair growth at these times are not fully understood, although it is felt that hormonal factors play a role.

Occasionally, excess facial hair can be caused by the use of certain medications. People taking the antihypertensive agent minoxidil often experience pronounced increased facial hair growth. As a matter of fact, doctors are currently trying to capitalize on this hair growing potential and are evaluating minoxidil's use in lotion form for growing hair on balding areas of the scalp (See Chapter 16). Other drugs, such as the steroid stimulating hormone, corticotropin (ACTH), and systemic steroid medications, used for treating a wide variety of conditions, have also been related to excess hair growth, especially following long-term use.

Excess facial hair may also be a manifestation of more serious underlying glandular disturbances. Glandular disorders of the ovaries, adrenal glands, or pituitary gland all may be causes of hirsutism. Medical attention should be sought if you experience a relatively sudden increase in the amount and coarseness of your body or facial hair, especially in areas where you did not have much hair before. You should also be concerned if you find excess hair growing upward from the pubic area toward the waist in a diamond-shaped pattern, or if you notice that you need to shave your legs and underarms more frequently than before. The appearance of acne, unusual weight gain, irregular periods, deepening of the voice, and enlargement of the clitoris should also prompt you to seek medical attention. A woman can waste precious time dealing with the purely cosmetic aspects of an excess hair problem without realizing that she really needs a thorough medical work-up. In fact, unless the underlying medical problem receives prompt attention, the excess hair problem will continue to worsen.

The remainder of this chapter will be devoted to the various chemical and mechanical ways you can deal with a problem of excess facial hair, once you have been assured that you have no serious underlying medical conditions.

MECHANICAL METHODS

Pumicing, Tweezing, and Shaving

Pumice stones, which may be purchased quite inexpensively in almost any drugstore, can be useful for removing fine facial hairs. They are made from a kind of volcanic rock that has been crushed into powder form and then pressed into various shapes and textures. Pumice stones are abrasive materials used for a variety of purposes. Coarser pumice stones are used for sanding down calluses or removing scaliness on the feet. Finer pumice stones are more suitable for rubbing and wearing away unwanted hairs. Of course, hairs removed in this way will regrow and you must periodically repeat the pumicing. When using a pumice stone for hair removal, you must take care not to rub too vigorously, for in your zeal you might also overly irritate or abrade the underlying skin. After pumicing, you should apply a thick emollient lotion to soothe your skin. As a rule, while safe and simple, the pumice method can be quite time-consuming, and is not particularly effective for removing coarser hairs.

Depilatory (hair-removing) gloves are a variation of the pumice method. These gloves are made of a fine sandpaper, which is shaped into the form of a mitten. With depilatory gloves, stubble can be smoothed away with a gentle circular motion. This procedure can be relatively quick and non-irritating. If needed, it may even be performed several times per day. Again, gentle abrasion is the key to keeping skin irritation to a minimum.

Tweezing or plucking is a very effective means for temporarily removing unwanted hairs. Unfortunately, as many of you already know, tweezing is very uncomfortable, sometimes even eye-wateringly painful. The number of hairs that can be tweezed at any time is limited only by how much discomfort you can stand at one time. That's not all. Plucking may occasionally result in the development of troublesome pustules around the plucked sites. Hair removal by plucking is only temporary, since each pluck will usually initiate a growing cycle for a new hair to replace the one that was removed. Contrary to a popular fear, tweezing of the hairs in a mole does not cause cancer. Occasionally, however, the mole will become irritated. For that reason cutting the hairs flush with the surface of the mole would be preferable to tweezing. While you really can't consider tweezing a permanent method of hair removal, repeated tweezing of the same hairs can sometimes damage the roots of those hairs so badly it can prevent them from ever regrowing—a kind of desirable traction alopecia.

Women shudder at the thought of shaving their faces. The decidedly masculine association of shaving the beard and the feeling of "loss" of femininity can be difficult to cope with. To add to the distress, there is a common misconception that once any area is shaved, the hair there will regrow not only more rapidly from that point on, but will be thicker and coarser thereafter. Happily, this is simply not so.

A typical hair shaft, which is normally wider in the middle and tapered at the end, will appear thicker and coarser when cut across at the skin surface. This is precisely because the hair has been cut at its widest point, rather than at its narrower end. Shaving causes no permanent change in your hair, nor will the hair regrow any faster afterward. And shaving does have several advantages. It is quick, painless, and effective. Stubble shadow can be covered with a suitable foundation makeup. To minimize unsightly and uncomfortable shaving nicks and cuts, the area to be shaved should be thoroughly wet and richly lathered. If an electric shaver is used, your skin should be completely dry. However, for a smoother closer shave, a razor is generally best.

Waxing and "Zipping"

Wax epilation, or simply, waxing, is a relatively unpopular procedure for temporary hair removal. Although home preparations do exist, waxing is most often done in professional salons. The area of the face that is most commonly waxed is the upper lip.

Waxing consists of thinly applying heated, melted wax to your skin, allowing it to cool and solidify to imbed the hairs, and then stripping it off in the direction of hair growth from the skin surface. In its essentials, waxing really amounts to a form of widespread plucking; the imbedded, unwanted hairs are actually pulled out *en masse*, rather than individually plucked. As with plucking, since individual hairs are pulled out at their root, regrowth takes a relatively long time, roughly six to eight weeks. Skin irritation, either from the heat or the plucking, is not uncommon.

Before having waxing done, hairs must be allowed to grow sufficiently long to ensure that they become tightly imbedded in the wax. Because of this the excess facial hair often becomes quite visible about one week before the next waxing. For some women, this can be a source of considerable embarrassment.

Zipping is basically the same procedure as waxing, except for the use of a cloth strip. After the heated wax is placed on the skin, a cloth strip is used to cover it. When the wax solidifies, the cloth strip is pulled ("zipped") away in the direction of hair growth, thereby pulling the unwanted hairs out by their roots. The advantages and disadvantages are the same as for waxing. The topical application of the female hormone estrogen has been added to the zipping procedure in hopes of achieving permanent hair removal. There is no scientific evidence, however, that the inclusion of estrogens has any beneficial effect at all.

Electrolysis

Until now I have described physical methods for temporarily removing facial hair. Electrolysis is the only method designed to *permanently* remove excess hair. It consists of sliding a very fine *epilating* (hair-removing), electric needle down the length of the hair shaft until it reaches the hair root. An electric current is then applied to the hair root in order to permanently destroy it.

Two methods of electrolysis are commonly employed. One method, which is used less often these days, employs a *galvanic* current. This causes water in your tissues to break up into electric charges, which in turn are responsible for destroying the hair roots. This process is correctly referred to as true electrolysis. A major drawback of galvanic electrolysis is that it is a relatively slow procedure in which fewer hairs can be treated during any one treatment session. This is why galvanic electrolysis is seldom used today. On the other hand, regrowth of hair after galvanic electrolysis occurs less often than with electrocoagulation, which will be discussed next.

Electrocoagulation is a more frequently used method of "electrolysis." It involves the use of a high-frequency electric current to generate tissue-destroying heat. Although electrocoagulation technically differs from true galvanic electrolysis, it is also commonly referred to as electrolysis. However, electrocoagulation is faster, and many more hairs can be removed per session. However, hair regrowth with high-frequency electrocoagulation occurs more frequently than with true electrolysis.

Electrolysis of either kind, even when it is limited to removing facial hair, has several drawbacks. In general, treatment takes a long time, is expensive, and is often painful. Inflammation around hair follicles (folliculitis), acne flare-ups, scarring, and spotty post-treatment pigmentation are common complications. In addition, treatment sessions may last thirty minutes and may be required once to twice weekly for several weeks, months, or, in more extensive cases, even several years.

In general, I recommend that people seek only experienced, and preferably licensed or certified, electrologists. Unfortunately, standards for the training and licensing of electrologists vary widely from state to state. A satisfactory cosmetic result depends upon the skill of the individual electrologist. Skill is needed to be able to slide the epilating needle down the hair shaft at the proper angle to reach the hair root. If the root is missed, the hair will grow back. Several hundred hairs can be treated per session. A good result requires that just the right amount of electric current be applied for the shortest time to destroy only the hair bulb. Leaving the current on for too long or applying too high a current can result in unnecessary pain and surrounding tissue damage, which can lead to hyperpigmentation or scarring. With either method of electrolysis, even in the best of hands, regrowth of individual hairs occurs about 40 precent of the time. This is often the most frustrating aspect of undergoing electrolysis. A reserve of patience is a must for anyone who opts for this method of hair removal.

Recently, newer and more flexible epilating needles have been devised that permit the epilating needle to more easily slide down even the most curved hair follicles right to the hairbulb. In addition, these special needles are insulated along their length so that the electrical current concentrates at the tip of the needle only, rather than along its entire length. By exposing only the hairbulb to the electric current in this fashion, there is less pain and less risk of scarring. Unfortunately, flexible, insulated epilating needles have only recently been introduced and are not widely available as yet.

If you choose electrolysis for hair removal, make certain that your electrologist pays careful attention to hygiene. Hepatitis and possibly even AIDS transmission are potential hazards of using contaminated needles. Furthermore, you shouldn't have a treatment session if you have an active herpes infection on your lips (cold sore, fever blister), since the herpes virus may be spread by contamination to other areas of your face. Finally, should you wish electrolysis for the removal of hairs growing from a mole, it would be advisable to consult a dermatologist first in order to make certain that the mole is otherwise entirely normal. In fact, most electrologists that I know are reluctant to remove hair from any mole unless a dermatologist has given a prior okay. For this reason, I generally perform the electrolysis on hairy moles myself. An added plus: Following electrolysis, many moles shrink considerably in size.

Home Electrolysis

Home electrolysis units can sometimes be of value for some women, particularly those having relatively few hairs to remove. These units are generally true galvanic electrolysis units and therefore work relatively slowly. Individual hairs may require as much as forty-five seconds of current to be destroyed. This limits the number of hairs that can reasonably be treated to about forty to fifty hairs per hour.

Home electrolysis units are typically battery-powered, hand-held units. PERMATWEEZ, produced by General Medical Company, Los Angeles, California, has a purportedly self-correcting spring action mechanism so that when its round-ended needle is introduced into the pore, it springs down to the hairbulb. The blunt tip of the needle has been specially designed to be too large to penetrate normal skin. Even an untrained individual can become quite successful in using this type of unit for most areas of the body after only a few practice sessions.

It takes practice to properly use home electrolysis units on your face, largely because you have to do it with a mirror and each movement you actually make becomes reversed in the mirror. Thus, if you move the unit to your right, it will appear to be moving to the left in the mirror. In addition, older or infirm individuals may have particular difficulty holding up the electrolysis unit for the thirty to forty-five seconds usually required to treat each hair.

Finally, a newly publicized method of hair removal utilizing radio frequency waves has been introduced. Instead of employing electricity or heat for hair removal, this method uses radio frequency waves which are transmitted down to the hair root through a specially designed tweezer. The drawbacks of electrolysis, namely pain, scarring, and hyperpigmentation, are supposed to be eliminated by this process. Whether this method will actually prove any better than conventional methods of electrolysis remains to be seen.

CHEMICAL METHODS

Bleaching

Bleaching the hair to make it less obvious is one of the simplest, most inexpensive, and painless ways of dealing with excess hair.

Bleaching generally works better if you have light colored skin. The less the contrast between the color of the bleached hairs and the color of your skin, the better. Bleaching preparations usually contain 6 percent hydrogen peroxide, often referred to as 20 volume hydrogen peroxide. Six percent hydrogen peroxide may even be used by itself. However, the peroxide is frequently combined with an alkali, usually ammonia, which helps the peroxide to bleach more effectively and intensely.

Although commercial hair bleaching products are available, you can easily prepare a homemade bleaching solution by simply adding ten to twenty drops of regular household ammonia to one fluid ounce of fresh 6 percent hydrogen peroxide. The peroxide must be fresh or bleaching will be inadequate. Once applied, the bleaching solution should be left in place for about thirty minutes and then thoroughly rinsed off with cool water. You should apply a good moisturizer to your skin following bleaching to minimize skin irritation. If you wish further lightening, repeat the bleaching procedure forty-eight hours later. Before bleaching an entire area, however, apply a small amount of bleaching solution to a tiny test area and leave it in place for thirty minutes. If no irritation develops, you may proceed to bleach the entire desired area.

Chemical Depilatories
(Hair Removers)

Chemical depilatories work by breaking down the sulfur bonds that hold the proteins in your hair together. They reduce the unwanted hairs to a jelly-like mass, which you can then easily wipe away. Chemical depilatories work above and slightly below the surface of your skin. They are available in creams, lotions, and spray foams and generally contain either sulfides or thioglycollates. Since your hair and skin are composed of similar chemicals, depilatories, especially if you don't carefully follow the directions, are notorious for irritating the skin. In general, depilatories should not be left in place for more than five minutes. Carefully read the product label to be sure that you are using a product specifically formulated for removal of facial hair. I strongly advise that you try a small amount of the depilatory on a test area before applying it to a large area.

Sulfides are the most effective depilatory ingredients. Unfortunately, they can be highly irritating. They also tend to have a rather unpleasant "rotten-eggs"-like odor. Thioglycollates are somewhat less effective, and must be kept on longer, but are usually less irritating and do not generate a foul odor. Because of the potential for irritation, follow all product label instructions very carefully and familiarize yourself with the procedure before you start.

A word of caution: The use of X-ray therapy for hair removal is obsolete and should be condemned. While forbidden by state law in many areas of the country, this procedure may occasionally still be found performed by untrained, nonmedical quacks. X-ray-induced cancer may occur at X-ray treatment sites many years after the initial treatments.

Finally, if you have a problem with excess facial hair, it is important for you to realize that you are not alone. Many other perfectly normal women are likewise affected. Further, there are a variety of effective ways for dealing with this problem. It is also important for you to keep in mind that as we continue to learn more about hair growth and hair physiology, newer, more effective ways of dealing with this troubling problem will appear on the horizon.

9

Trouble-Free Shaving

In the last chapter, I briefly touched upon shaving as a means for some women to manage excessive facial hair. Most men, however, have to deal with shaving on a daily basis. For some men, particularly those whose jobs require them to be clean shaven, shaving can sometimes lead to special facial and neck problems. For most men, however, trouble-free shaving simply requires knowing some basic facts about safety razors vs. electric shavers, preshave products, shaving preparations, and after-shave products.

RAZORS VS. ELECTRIC SHAVERS

The most common question patients ask me about shaving is: Which gives the *best* shave, a razor blade or an electric shaver? Some evidence exists that electric shavers don't give as close or uniform a shave as razors do. Moreover, the cut ends of your hairs, the stubble, are more likely to be left jagged and frayed following shaving with an electric shaver.

Razor blades come in a variety of types: the straightedge, which the barber uses, and several kinds of safety razors—the old style, loose, double-edge razors, disposable razors and single and twin blade injectable cartridge razors. Almost all razor blades today are made of stainless steel and are good for about ten shaves per blade, depending upon how heavy the beard is. The choice of blade is a matter of personal preference. Just about any one of them is capable of giving a safe, close shave. Razors referred to as safety razors are made in such a way that you cannot seriously cut yourself with them while shaving properly. Even when they are improperly used, not enough of the blade is exposed to do any more harm than simply nicking the skin. By contrast, straightedge razors are basically very sharp knives and have the potential for serious injury if used improperly.

For the most part, the least expensive kinds of safety razors will give you as good a shave as the more expensive varieties. Choice then becomes a matter of convenience, cost, and personal preference. The razor apparatus should feel comfortable in your hand and should be easily maneuverable across the specific contours of your face. In dealing with certain special facial conditions, however, disposable razors can be particularly useful. (Special shaving situations are covered at the end of this chapter.)

Electric shavers basically come in two types of design, the foil head and the rotary head. The foil head, the most common variety, consists of a thin, flexible screen under which the cutting head moves back and forth. The rotary head shavers consist of spring-mounted guards that surmount the cutters. Some shavers have a number of different settings that permit you to raise or lower the shaver's cutting head(s) to regulate the closeness of the shave. Such adjustable electric shavers may be particularly useful for individuals with special facial problems.

Nevertheless, all the foregoing information still doesn't really answer the basic question, namely: Which shaving method, razor or electric shaver, gives you the best shave? So far, you only know that the razor method of shaving is generally felt to cut hairs closer and smoother. *The question about the best shaving method can only be answered by you.* The answer will depend upon several factors—your skin type, the type of hair you have, the required frequency of shaving, the coexistence of other skin conditions or problems, and personal preferences. It is interesting that in most other Westernized industrial nations, between 50 and 75 percent of men routinely use electric shavers. By contrast, only about 25 percent of American men (and less than 50 percent of women) prefer electric shavers. In general, if you have otherwise normal skin, the thicker your facial hair and the more dense your beard, the more likely you will need a razor blade to give you an adequately close shave. On the other hand, if you have sensitive skin or an acne condition, you may be better off using an electric shaver.

If you opt to shave with a razor blade, make certain that you adequately moisten and soften your beard *before* shaving to prevent nicks and cuts. If you should decide that an electric shaver would best suit your needs, look for one that gives you the closeness of shave you desire without excessively pulling or nicking your skin. Finally, no one method of shaving is best for everyone. In the final analysis, it takes a little trial and error to find out which shaving method is *right for you.*

PRESHAVE PRODUCTS

Most preshave products that are currently available are largely intended for use before electric shaving. However, preshave products for razor shaving are also available. Preshave products of both kinds have been developed to make shaving easier, faster, less uncomfortable, and less irritating to the skin.

Preshave products for use before wet shaving are designed to wet your beard and soften the hairs before the application of the shaving cream. These products generally contain a soap or synthetic detergent, as well as lubricants. The soap or detergent is supposed to degrease the hairs so that the hairs may then more easily absorb water, swell, and stiffen. Synthetic detergents, mentioned in Chapter 1, are preferable for use in hard water areas because they lather better and leave no soap scum residue on your beard and skin.

In general, you can achieve the same moistening effects without the use of a preshave by thoroughly wetting or washing your face with warm water before shaving. Then, apply your regular shaving preparation and let it remain in contact with your skin for about two to three minutes. If the shaving cream begins to dry, you can add a little more warm water. Finally, reapply more shaving cream right before you begin shaving.

Pre-electric shave products are designed to do just the opposite of preshave products for wet razor shaving. Rather than moistening and softening your beard, these products are intended to dry and stiffen the hairs. The ideal preshave product for electric shaving should be astringent (drying), mildly acidic, quick drying, nonirritating, and noncorrosive to the shaving head of the electric razor.

Some brands of preshave preparations tend to be more oily than astringent. In those cases, the product is intended more for lubricating the skin to prevent drag than it is for stiffening the hairs of the beard. In the final analysis, for most individuals, a specific pre-electric shave product is really not necessary. Simply apply powder sparingly to your face before electric shaving, and you will get the needed dryness to shave smoothly and comfortably.

SHAVING PREPARATIONS
FOR WET SHAVING
(RAZOR SHAVING)

In addition to the use of plain soap, a number of different types of wet shaving preparations are commercially available. These include lather creams, aerosol foams and gels, and brushless shaving creams. Whiskers, which are composed of the same protein, keratin, found in skin, are hard and stiff when dry and, without proper moisturization, it would generally require a good deal of pressure to cut them with a razor. The more pressure you need to use to shave, the more likely your face will become nicked, scratched, or irritated. All shaving preparations are intended to prevent shaving "burn" (chapped or scratched skin) by moistening and softening your whiskers and holding them sufficiently upright to permit closer, more trouble-free razor shaving.

At the present time, aerosol preparations, which number about two dozen, account for about 95 percent of the total market. With the exception of the brushless shaving products, all other wet shaving formulations fundamentally contain non-irritating, lather-producing soaps or detergents. However, it's really the water that softens your beard, not the detergent. Water remains the most effective beard softener, but the soaps or detergents in shaving preparations, like those in preshave lotions, remove the protective oily film from your whiskers and permit the hairs to better absorb the water.

Soaps, Lather Shaving Creams, and Aerosols

Plain soap was the prototype of shaving preparations. While soaps lather well, in order to generate sufficient lather for shaving they have to be lathered thoroughly in a mug and applied with a brush. Soaps are rarely used today for that reason. Lather shaving creams are also composed of soaps. However, lubricating oils, water-retaining humectants, and foam stabilizers have been added to these products to make them more efficient than plain soap. As their name implies, lather shaving creams must still be lathered in a mug and applied with a brush in order to produce enough lather. On the market for years, these preparations still enjoy a modest popularity.

As mentioned earlier, aerosol shaving preparations, either creams or gels, remain the most popular. The basic ingredients in these products differ little from those contained in lather creams. Aerosols are basically lotions to which propellants are added to permit a foamy, lathered discharge from the can. In general, the shave you get using aerosols is similar to the kind you get using ordinary lather creams. The main advantage of aerosols is their ease of application. Aerosols have all the pluses of lather creams, without the need for mugs and brushes. It is no doubt this convenience that accounts for the enormous popularity of aerosol shaving preparations over the past two decades.

Most aerosol products appear to be equally effective and equally economical. Many brands of aerosol shaving products only cost between one-half and one cent per shave—a pretty reasonable deal considering the inflationary times in which we live.

Heat accelerates the absorption of moisture into the whiskers. In addition, as anyone who has sat in a barber's chair and had a hot towel placed on their face can tell you, warm water on the face, like hot baths and showers, can be quite relaxing and stress-reducing. For these reasons, hot-lather shaving creams have also enjoyed some measure of popularity. In some products, the foam heats itself right on your face. (A hydrogen peroxide reaction with other ingredients in the foam accounts for the heat generated.)

Nevertheless, hot-lather shaving preparations really do not offer any significant shaving advantages over what you can achieve by thoroughly moistening your face with warm water before shaving. However, these shaving preparations do offer convenience, while providing some of you with a soothing shaving experience. Hot preparations generally cost about three to six times as much per shave (between two cents and three cents) as regular shaving creams, but if that's what it takes to pamper yourself, I have no basic objections to your using them.

Brushless Shaving Creams

Brushless shaving preparations, which contain little or no soap or detergent, do not lather. They are generally composed of an oil-in-water vanishing cream base, to which surfactants and humectants (see Chapter 4) have been added. The oil in the moisturizing cream base is deposited upon the skin and remains on the skin after shaving. This lubrication is supposed not only to soften the skin, but to minimize after-shave irritation.

Unfortunately, brushless shaving creams generally take longer than lather creams to moisturize the beard. For that reason, they should be allowed to remain in contact with your beard for several minutes before shaving. Alternatively, they may be applied after the use of a wet shave, preshave lotion, or following a thorough moistening or washing of your skin with warm water. Brushless shaving products are the most lubricating of all wet shaving products and are particularly useful for people with dry or sensitive skin. Brushless shaving creams are also a travel convenience because you don't need to pack a shaving mug and brush, and you don't have to worry about the shaving cream spraying out of the aerosol can during luggage handling.

AFTER-SHAVE PRODUCTS

After-shave products, as their name clearly suggests, are meant to be used after you finish shaving. They may be used after razor or electric shaving. Most after-shave products are intended to refresh your face and soothe shaving discomfort. On the other hand, men's colognes, which frequently are suggested for after-shave use, are intended primarily for their fragrance.

Several types of after-shave products are commonly available: after-shave lotions, refreshers, or skin bracers. The different names imply different ingredient compositions or functions. In fact, all of these products actually differ little in their basic ingredient makeup, although the proportions may vary. All three are largely composed of alcohol, water, and fragrance. Skin bracers and refreshers generally have a higher alcohol content than after-shave lotions, and may also be used for the rest of the body. After-shave lotions are generally intended for after-shave, facial use only. Finally, colognes, which are a blend of fragrances, are usually less strongly scented than after-shave lotions, refreshers, or skin bracers, and as mentioned earlier are sold for their fragrance esthetics, rather than for any after-shave comfort purposes.

Unless you particularly enjoy the feel or scent of after-shave preparations, they really are not necessary. In fact, if you have nicked or abraded your skin during shaving, they can sting quite a bit when you first put them on. Otherwise, I have no particular objection to them. The best way to ensure after-shave comfort is to shave properly.

SPECIAL
SHAVING PROBLEMS

Flat Warts (Verruca Plana)
and Shaving

All true warts are benign, infectious growths caused by virus members of the family known as the *human papilloma viruses*. Warts are not to be confused with a variety of other growths, moles, or "beauty marks" that can be found on the face (Chapter 12).

Flat warts are a variety of wart that commonly affect the face. They generally appear as small, flat, mostly flesh-colored to pinkish, opaque bumps. If you think you have them, you should consult a dermatologist to have them removed because warts tend to spread, particularly within the beard area of actively shaving men. In fact, it is the shaving process itself that helps to spread wart viruses from one part of the face to another, where they take hold within microscopic shaving nicks and scratches. I have had occasion to treat men who have had literally hundreds of warts present throughout the beard areas of their face and neck, the result of ignoring their problem for several weeks or months.

When the warts have become numerous, treatment usually requires several sessions spanning a period of several weeks. Since the spread of these viruses is in part related to the act of shaving, when you first notice them, and while you are undergoing treatments, you should follow some simple rules. If you use a razor, change blades between shaves. Do not use the same blade twice. Always shave the noninvolved areas first. If you shave in the opposite order, namely the infected areas first, you risk spreading the virus to previously noncontaminated areas. Remember, shave the wart areas last.

If you use an electric razor, clean the cutters and foil screens before each use with a gauze pad saturated with alcohol. Do not use a cotton pledget, since the fibers may shred on to the shaving apparatus. Here, too, as with razor shaving, shave the affected areas last.

Ingrown Beard Hairs
(Pseudofolliculitis Barbae)

Ingrown beard hairs or *pseudofolliculitis barbae* are a minor, but nonetheless quite troubling skin condition which affects many white men and the majority of black men. The condition results from the penetration of the hair follicle wall, or more commonly, the penetration of the skin adjacent to the hair follicle by sharpened, incurving beard hairs. This cutting results in infection and inflammation, as implied by its suffix, "itis," meaning inflammation. The reason it is called *pseudo*folliculitis is because the inflammation does not truly affect the hair follicle, but the area around it.

Ingrown beard hairs appear to result from a familial or racial tendency for thick, coarse, curly hair. Ordinarily, for most people with straighter hair, hairs which have retracted slightly below the surface following a close shave usually grow straight out again through their regular pore opening at the skin surface. For people with a tendency for ingrown beard hairs, the tight curve of the cut hair may angle away from the pore opening from which it retracted, and, as it regrows, the hair may then pierce the skin to the side of the pore like a knife, causing inflammation.

Ingrown beard hairs appear like tiny pimples or pustules.

They may be very painful and can bleed easily. After they resolve, areas of ingrown hair may remain temporarily or even permanently discolored (usually darkened), or even permanently scarred. The neck is usually particularly affected.

If you suffer from this condition, the most consistently effective approach you can take is not to shave. Within about one month after allowing your beard to grow, you will find that your problem is largely gone. In other words, all the embedded hairs will have sprung out in that time. If shaving is a must, you might try allowing your beard to grow out during an extended vacation. Once most of the problem has been resolved, you can then follow the hair removing methods described below.

If you use a razor blade, be sure to soak and moisten your whiskers thoroughly before shaving. You might precede shaving by making an effort to tease out with a fine needle (precleaned with alcohol) any hairs that are lying horizontally or are embedded near the surface. You might also try using an abrasive, web-polyester sponge, such as a BUF PUF sponge, or even a toothbrush to dislodge hairs which are just beginning to embed themselves.

Always change your blades frequently to ensure a sharp, less angulated cut. A jagged edge to the stubble can make the problem worse. Do not stretch your skin while shaving; this will make the cut closer or even slightly below the pore surface, promoting retraction of the whiskers below the surface—just what you don't want. Shave with the grain of the whiskers, not against it, since shaving against the grain will result in a closer shave. It is better to shave less closely and more frequently.

If you use an electric shaver, purchase one with multiple settings and regulate the setting for the lightest shave possible. Alternatively, you might try using hair clippers to trim your whiskers. Hair clippers usually do not cut closely enough to aggravate the ingrown hair problem. If hair clipping alone does not give you enough of a clean-shaven look (and it usually doesn't), you might try alternating shaving with clipping the beard hairs.

The use of chemical depilatories and electrolysis has already been discussed in the last chapter. While chemical depilatories do a satisfactory job of hair removal and can be quite useful in dealing with the problem of ingrown beard hairs, they are often too irritating to use on a daily basis. However, depilatories may be used on a rotational basis every few days to supplement the other methods of hair removal already mentioned.

Electrolysis remains the only true cure for ingrown beard hairs. When electrolysis is neither feasible nor desirable, and the other methods of hair removal already described have provided only marginal benefit, you should consult a dermatologist. The dermatologist has at his or her disposal a variety of prescription topical antibiotics and anti-inflammatories, which in many cases can help to ameliorate the problem.

Acne

Daily shaving can be a difficult problem for the person suffering from facial acne. In many cases, the skin is already sore and inflamed, and shaving only makes it more so. Fragile pimples and pustules can be nicked or ruptured during shaving, and oozing and bleeding can result. In addition, the use of soap or detergent-containing shaving products may contribute to excessive drying of the skin, making the application of topical anti-acne medications too uncomfortable to tolerate. This is because anti-acne topicals are frequently themselves slightly over-drying. On the other hand, brushless shaving creams intended to moisturize sensitive skin may leave the skin too oily for use by acne sufferers. Finally, the mechanical pulling and pushing of the razor or shaver on the skin may rupture hidden whiteheads below the surface and further aggravate the acne problem.

In general, I recommend adjustable-setting electric razors for my patients with acne. The setting should be for the lightest shave possible. The lighter the setting (and hence, the less close the shave that you get with it), the less irritating it will be to already irritated, sensitive skin. With electric shavers, many people find that bleeding from nicking and cutting is also less of a problem than with razor shaving. Once again, as with the ingrown beard hair problem, it is still better to shave gently and more frequently than more closely and less frequently. By shaving with an electric shaver, you also need not use a potentially overly drying shaving product, or an overly oily brushless shaving cream. At the same time, you should, of course, be doing something to take care of your acne problem. Chapters 7 and 15 cover what you and your doctor can do to control acne.

10

Dealing with Hair Loss

For many women, concern about hair loss may put them in a state of near-panic. Most women who experience loss of hair have visions of losing all their hair and looking like a bald man. Fortunately, this type of balding in women is rare. However, the panic and concern are understandable. Straight hair can be made curly, dark hair light, and vice-versa, but a bald head cannot usually be made to re-grow hair, and this is what frightens anyone experiencing hair thinning or loss. By playing on this fear, some unethical manufacturers and advertisers are able to sell millions of dollars' worth of useless "hair-growing" or "hair-loss-preventing" concoctions.

There are many causes of hair thinning and hair loss. Some conditions affect the growing hair root, some do not. Some types of hair loss are reversible; unhappily, many are not. Finally, there are situations that appear to be true hair loss, but really are not. Common causes of hair thinning and hair loss, proven methods for preventing some kinds of hair loss, and ways you can deal with permanent hair loss are the subjects of this chapter. Specific medical conditions or drugs that can lead to temporary or permanent hair loss, and their treatments, will be discussed in Chapter 16.

REVERSIBLE HAIR LOSS

Thin hair and *hair breakage* are conditions that are not really true hair loss problems. For the most part, thin hair is an inherited trait, like hair color. As I mentioned in Chapter 5, blond hair is the thinnest type of hair, red hair the thickest. A full head of blond hair must contain roughly forty thousand more hairs than a full head of red hair in order to give an equal impression of fullness. Other than using hair dyes, which either coat or swell your hairs depending upon whether you use temporary or permanent dyes, or through the use of protein conditioners and body builders, there is no way to change the pattern of growth of hair follicles to produce thicker hair.

Hair breakage is another condition that can give the impression, however false, of being a true hair loss problem. In fact, there is really nothing wrong with the hair root, the growing area of the hair. Hair breakage results from damage to the hair shafts caused by excessive bleaching, frequent permanent-waving, or straightening. These processes can render hair brittle, fragile, and unable to withstand normal daily hair care manipulations, such as combing, brushing, and blow-drying. If many hairs break, especially near the surface, a condition resembling true hair loss can result. However, since no permanent hair loss actually occurs, simply stopping all bleaching and waving for several months is usually all that is necessary to allow your hair to return to normal. In the meantime, the continued use of conditioners to "thicken," moisturize, and untangle the hair can also be helpful.

Individuals who habitually twirl, bite, or chew on their hair may temporarily damage their hair. The damage is purely mechanical trauma to the hair shafts. In these cases, hair fragility and breakage result solely from overmanipulation. Making the person aware of the habit is usually enough to stop it. Once the habit is stopped, the hair grows back normally.

Traction Alopecia (Baldness)

The word *traction* means pulling, tugging, or tension, and the phrase *traction alopecia* means hair loss resulting from excessive tension on hair roots. The frequent use of tightly wound rollers, or such tightly pulled hair styles as ponytails, pigtails, hair-plaiting, "corn-rowing," and braiding have all been known to lead to traction alopecia. Traction alopecia usually results in hair loss and hair breakage at the front and sides of the scalp where tension on the hair roots is generally the greatest. The injury to the roots is frequently reversible within several months if the rollers or tension-producing styles are stopped. However, if these styling practices are continued, or too frequently repeated, permanent and irreversible hair loss may result.

Stress-Related Hair Loss
Telogen Effluvium

At any one time, in a normal head of hair, approximately 85 percent of all hairs are actively growing and are called *anagen* hairs. The remaining 15 percent are in a resting stage and are called *telogen* hairs. Telogen hairs are gradually shed and, after a short time, are replaced by new anagen hairs.

Occasionally, during times of particular physical or emotional stress, many more hairs may become prematurely shifted into the resting phase and then shed *en masse*. Stresses on the body, such as a prolonged high fever, childbirth, surgery, crash dieting, and bereavement have been associated with pronounced telogen hair loss, which generally doesn't begin right away. Instead, telogen hair loss usually occurs about four to eight weeks after the particular stress has actually passed.

The amount of hair loss can be frightening. It may begin to fall out in large clumps and batches, and distressing amounts of hair may be found on the pillow or come out while combing or brushing. It may continue to the point where over 40 percent of the normal number of scalp hairs are lost, at which point the loss is quite noticeable. Telogen hair loss usually continues for several weeks before tapering off. If the original stress has been eliminated, hair will usually begin to grow back normally within a few weeks. However, since hair only grows about a half inch per month, noticeable improvement generally takes at least six months. Patience, combined with gentle, routine hair and scalp care and a "tincture of time," are the most effective therapies for telogen hair loss. Unfortunately, no drug can speed the process of regrowth. If hair loss persists, a dermatologist should be consulted.

IRREVERSIBLE HAIR LOSS

Menopausal Hair Loss

With the passage of time, the rate of hair loss gradually begins to exceed the rate of new growth. It would be very rare indeed to see a woman in her eighties with as much hair as she had in her twenties. Hair thinning may become particularly noticeable after menopause and, like increased hair growth on the upper lip and chin which may occur at about the same time, probably is related to hormonal changes.

Other than maintaining normal hair and scalp care, little can be done for this almost universal process of gradual hair loss. The use of various types of hormone creams to reverse it has been tried without much success. In fact, these creams may even be harmful, depending upon which hormones are used and how much of them are absorbed through the skin into the general circulation.

Female Pattern Baldness
(Female Androgenetic Alopecia)

Female *androgenetic alopecia*, or female pattern baldness, is a less well-recognized form of permanent hair loss. Most of us

are familiar with the usual pattern of male balding, which generally takes the form of hair loss at the temples and the crown,
and may begin in a hereditarily predisposed man as early as his
late teens or early twenties. Many of you may have been un-
aware that hereditarily predisposed women, too, have a characteristic pattern of balding. Female pattern hair loss generally
takes the form of a diffuse hair loss across the entire top of the
scalp. Because it doesn't occur at the temples, and because
feminine hair styling is often effectively used by those with the
problem to cover balding areas, female pattern hair loss is less
easily spotted by outsiders. This accounts in large measure for
why fewer people are aware of the existence of female pattern
baldness, and why many women with a hair loss problem complain to me that they have never seen anyone else with the
same problem.

Three main factors are felt to be responsible for balding in
both men and women: heredity, age, and male hormones.
(Women normally have approximately two-thirds as much
male hormone as men.) While it seems that these otherwise
healthy men and women are not producing an excess of male
hormone, it is believed that their hair follicles are more sensitive to the amount of male hormone they *do* produce, and this
heightened sensitivity to male hormone is considered to be
responsible for hair loss.

A number of popular misconceptions about male and female
pattern balding exist. Balding is *not* caused by the use of tight
hats, headbands, or wigs. The normal scalp has such a rich network of blood vessels that circulation of blood isn't really
affected by wearing constrictive headgear. Nor does frequent
or daily shampooing cause balding. Excessive cleansing can
often make your hair dry, brittle, and more fragile, resulting in
hair breakage, and this can make your hair appear sparser, but
no permanent damage is really done.

Persistently oily hair and severe dandruff do *not* cause hair
loss or balding. Occasionally, a dandruffy scalp inflammation
(seborrheic dermatitis) may be so severe that some resting hairs

are shed prematurely, giving the impression that hair loss has worsened. However, resting hairs are constantly being replaced by new, normal growing hairs and no overall change actually occurs. Finally, diet plays *no* role in ordinary hereditary hair loss. Any additional intake of vitamins, minerals, or other foods, above what is necessary to maintain a balanced diet, will have no effect on preventing or reversing hereditary baldness.

If your parents, grandparents, aunts, uncles, brothers, or sisters have experienced hair loss with aging, it indicates that a hereditary susceptibility for hair thinning and hair loss exists in your family. Some people believe that the trait for baldness is inherited from the father only; in fact, this trait can be inherited from *either* parent. The trait can also skip generations and spare many members of a particular family.

Hereditary hair loss follows a regular pattern in men and women. In the balding areas, hair follicles become progressively smaller and have shorter growing periods. The hairs themselves become progressively thinner, lighter in color, and shorter in length. Finally, the hair follicles in balding areas may completely shrivel up and produce only a fine, almost imperceptible, fuzz.

No miracle cures for baldness are yet available, although the research continues. Certainly no shampoos or nonprescription creams or ointments exist that can either prevent hair loss or restore lost hair. Any such claims are false. Not too long ago, a manufacturer of a hair product containing jojoba oil claimed that its product not only prevented hair loss, but could regrow hair. The claim was blatantly false and the company finally was forced to withdraw its product from the market (for hair-growing products), but by then it had already sold millions of dollars' worth of its product to unwary—and desperately hopeful—customers. A prescription lotion, minoxidil, which is currently under intensive investigation for its effects on hair-loss prevention and hair growth stimulation, will be discussed in Chapter 16.

HAIRWEAVING

Originally limited to dealing with male pattern baldness, hair-weaving has more recently been used successfully for dealing with female hair loss. Hairweaving is basically a procedure in which color- and texture-matched human hair is woven, braided, or knotted into your own natural hair. Your natural hair is used to anchor the newly woven hair in place. With this technique, even if you've lost a lot of hair, you can be "restored" to a full head of hair. Once in place, the woven hair can be cut and styled to your taste. Since your natural anchoring hairs continue to grow out, the hairweave gradually lifts away from your scalp and loosens every few weeks. Depending upon how fast the natural anchoring hairs grow, hairweave retightening may be needed every four to eight weeks.

As with almost any procedure, there are advantages and disadvantages to hairweaving. On the plus side, hairweaving involves no surgery, no cutting, no pain. The hairweave remains in place during exercise and swimming and feels entirely nat-ural. In trained hands, the cosmetic results of hairweaving can be excellent and quite gratifying.

On the negative side, the hairweaving method can be expen-sive. Depending upon the length of hair that is desired, the initial hairweaving sessions may total several hundred to well over a thousand dollars. Each weaving session generally takes about two hours. In addition, each retightening session, which also requires about two hours, may run between fifty and a hundred and fifty dollars. If, for example, you needed to return for retightening every six weeks, the yearly maintenance costs for hairweaving could run from four hundred to twelve hundred dollars. Moreover, shampooing and caring for your scalp and natural hair underneath a hair weave can be difficult. Finally, traction by a tight hairweave on your natural anchoring hairs can occasionally result in hair loss or breakage of the natural hair (a form of traction alopecia). Nevertheless, in the hands of a skilled and experienced professional, hairweaving can be a quick and psychologically satisfying means for dealing with a hair loss problem.

WIGS AND
AREA HAIRPIECES

Wigs and hairpieces are another alternative for people with thinning hair. Today, wigs and hairpieces are far more natural-looking than in past years. The selection is broad, and there are considerable differences in quality, cost, durability, and maintenance.

Custom-Made Wigs

Custom-made wigs are the highest quality wigs, and therefore the most expensive. They are handmade from human hair matched in color and texture to your natural hair and are fitted to your exact measurements. When well made, they look and feel natural. A custom-made wig usually requires three visits, for the purpose of taking your exact measurements, fitting the cap, and tinting, trimming, and styling the wig. Custom-made wigs can be dry-cleaned in a matter of minutes by dipping them in an evaporating solvent, which usually can be purchased from the wig-maker. After cleaning, the wig may be combed, brushed, or styled just like your normal hair. The colors of human-hair wigs may become bleached and faded by sun exposure, so color touch-ups may be periodically needed. The cost of a custom-wig may exceed twelve hundred dollars.

Customized ready-made wigs are a less expensive variety of the custom-made wig. These wigs average about five hundred dollars and are factory-produced human-hair wigs. The bases of these wigs are flexible enough to allow adjustment "customization" to fit specific head sizes. Like custom-made wigs, customized ready-made wigs can also be easily dry-cleaned and styled like normal hair.

Synthetic Wigs

Synthetic wigs, in which the "hairs" are made from synthetic fibers, come in two varieties—the *custom synthetic wig* and *ready-made* stock wig. Generally handmade, custom synthetic wigs allow you some individualization as far as measurement and color are concerned, but cost much less than custom-made wigs because they do not contain real human hair. These wigs can simply be washed in a mild shampoo. They are durable enough to be styled, blow-dried, and even curled using hot rollers. They usually cost between a hundred and fifty and five hundred dollars.

Ready-made stock wigs are the least expensive type of wig. They are mass-produced and mostly imported items that come in a variety of pre-set hairstyles and colors. These wigs tend to look somewhat unnatural and can be a little uncomfortable to wear. Ready-made stock wigs are usually made of synthetic fibers, but occasionally may be made from poor quality human hair. These wigs are easily cared for, and the better ones may even be styled or blow-dried. Their cost normally ranges from as low as twenty to as high as a hundred and fifty dollars. In my opinion, price is about the only thing that this kind of wig has going for it.

When purchasing a wig, besides paying attention to the types of fibers used, you should also examine the type of base used. In wig-making, the base is the material onto which the human hairs or synthetic fibers are anchored. Hard plastic bases tend to hold their shapes well. However, despite the ventilation holes in them, they may become uncomfortable, particularly when they are worn in warm and humid weather. Soft, synthetic fiber mesh bases are more comfortable in warmer and more humid climates because they can "breathe." However, mesh bases tend to stretch out of shape after a while. Lastly, there are transparent, synthetic meshes, called front laces, that extend slightly beyond the main bulk of the wig and need to be glued in place. While this type of base holds firmly, it requires more time to properly apply.

The Area Hairpiece

If you need to cover only a small patch of hair loss, you might find an *area hairpiece* preferable to a full wig. Any size, shape, and color can be customized to blend imperceptibly with your natural hair.

There is one final, but important, financial note about wigs and hairpieces. Wigs and hairpieces purchased specifically for hair loss or hair replacement reasons, rather than as fashion apparel, are considered *"medical hair prostheses"* by many health insurance companies. If you need a wig or hairpiece for medical reasons and your insurance carrier reimburses for these purposes, have your dermatologist write a refillable prescription for a "medical hair prosthesis." Furthermore, when used for hair loss purposes only, wigs and hair pieces may also constitute legitimate tax-deductible medical expenses. You should check, of course, with your lawyer about this matter.

11

To Facial or
Not to Facial?

Throughout Part I of this book, I have attempted to include, whenever possible, specific information about altogether bogus or only minimally useful skin care products or practices. I have stressed the message that "if something sounds too good to be true, it probably is *not* true." I would now like to touch upon another major area where you should exercise caution—the facial. Since my patients frequently ask whether they should be going for facials on a regular basis, and whether facials really do any good, I decided to devote a separate chapter to answering those questions. Much of what I say will apply equally to home facial rituals and professional salon facials.

FACIALS AND
FACIAL SALONS

Skin care salons are numerous and have been attempting to double their clientele by appealing to men as well as to women. It seems that almost every facial salon has its own regimens for cleaning, "nourishing," toning, stimulating, and rejuvenating your skin during the facial, as well as recommending cosmetics and skin care routines for home care between professional facial treatments. Costs for the basic facial, which usually lasts from one to two hours, range from about thirty to a hundred dollars per session. The cosmetics usually suggested by professional salon consultants for home use may cost you between eighty-five dollars and several hundred dollars more, depending upon the specific items purchased. You are frequently encouraged to buy a whole product line, being told that you need to use the entire "system" in order for it to really work. So, are facials worth it, or are they a waste of money?

In general, there are several factors which must be considered. One is a basic lack of uniformity in the training and experience of professional facial salon employees. Several years ago, during the course of one month, a correspondent for a leading magazine made the rounds of several of the largest and most famous facial salons in New York City. In each of the salons she visited she was told she had a completely different kind of skin. She was variously "diagnosed" as having "combination" skin, oily skin, normal skin, and dry skin. The correspondent was puzzled, and rightly so, by the completely different conclusions that each of these so-called skin care "experts" made about the same face. It disturbed me as well. One of my dermatologic colleagues, quoted in that same article, had the following comment to make on facial salon "diagnoses": "salons define normal so as to exclude most of the human race."

Now let's examine some of the more common home or salon facial techniques used to "treat" your skin and see if they stand up to scientific scrutiny. Some of these procedures include the use of vibrators, massagers, brushes, steam cleaning, facial saunas, heat lamps, and clay or gel masks. Such masks often contain collagen or herbals. You are frequently told, among other things, that these devices, methods, and ingredients are uniquely designed to deep-clean your skin, increase blood circulation, allow your pores to "breathe," "tighten" your pores, and restore collagen or other proteins and nutrients to your skin.

In fact, no product or device is able to get down to the

bottom of your pores and clean them. Pores do not have little muscles around them, so they cannot be exercised or treated in any other way to permanently tighten them up. Steaming can do little to get out whiteheads, pimples, or acne cysts since these types of blemishes no longer possess any pore openings to the surface to allow the trapped material within them to escape. These conditions may actually be worsened by steaming, precisely because the opening is closed or too small for any of the contents to be extracted. Even blackheads, which usually may be more easily cleaned out after steaming, will, as a rule, re-form shortly after the cleaning. Placing a warm, wet towel over your face for a few minutes will accomplish the same effects as steaming and facial saunas. Heat lamps also do little except warm the skin and perhaps make you feel better psychologically.

On the subject of masks, they, like astringents, brushes, and vigorous massaging or vibrating, slightly irritate your skin. Any type of irritation, for example, the kind of irritation you can get by rubbing or slapping your face vigorously, results in a slight swelling of the skin. It is precisely that swelling which gives that tighter, "healthier" look and feel to your skin that you frequently have after a facial. More specifically, it is the swelling that takes place around the surface rim of each of your pores that *temporarily* acts to make them appear smaller. The whole effect, however, only lasts at most a few hours; when the swelling finally subsides, you are right back to square one. Finally, as you learned in Chapter 2, your skin does not "eat up" or "drink in" collagen, herbs, vitamins, etc., whether applied in cream, lotion, or mask form. Nourishment comes from the blood vessels below the surface of the skin only.

The use of electric needles inserted below the skin to "treat" wrinkles is another procedure that has enjoyed a measure of popularity. Those that recommend the use of such electric devices claim that the small bursts of electric current applied restore the elasticity to the skin and rejuvenate skin cells. However, it is thought that any benefits observed from this method are due to irritation, this time below the skin surface and electrically induced. Once again, it is the swelling that most probably accounts for the *temporary* smoothing of the wrinkles. Shortly afterward, when the swelling subsides, the improvement disappears. The procedure itself is not without risk. Scarring and long-lasting, splotchy skin pigmentation have been known to occur, especially when too strong an electric current was applied.

In summary, for the reasons I have given here, I do not ordinarily recommend facials—either salon or home-based—to any of my patients with problem skin. Misrepresented or misunderstood claims for the benefits of facial treatments for certain conditions have occasionally even been responsible for delaying people from seeking proper expert medical advice when it was needed. For those of you with normal skin and ample expendable finances, facials can be a relaxing and indulging experience. If you are just such a person, I have no serious objections to your having a facial, so long as you know why you are having it and don't fall prey to advertising hype and sales pitches.

This chapter should not be miscontrued as a desire on my part to disparage either cosmetologists or beauticians. Indeed, they can play a crucial role in advising you about your options on such things as the proper choices of makeup and hairstyles to enhance your appearance. These specialists can also play a very important role in teaching you the best ways to apply makeup for your own special needs. Their role in making you look and feel better about yourself cannot and should not be minimized. I have often had the occasion to refer people to cosmeticians for their advice in these matters, particularly for their advice about the best hairstyles to camouflage thinning hair, or the best ways to cosmetically mask certain otherwise untreatable skin conditions. Clearly, to the person disturbed by problems such as these, the advice and services of a knowledgable cosmetician can be invaluable.

As a final comment for Part I, no one book can catalogue all the frauds, phony claims, and misrepresentations that exist. Even if it could, a new gimmick to sell merchandise seems to pop up every day. The best way to avoid wasting your money or time is to pay careful attention to what is being told to you, and to be aware of being overtly or subtly manipulated by advertising and salespeople. When you hear about some "miraculous" product, cure, treatment, method, or system, you should immediately think: Who says so? How did they prove it? If you can't get satisfactory answers to these questions, don't do it, or don't buy it!

PART II

WHAT YOUR DOCTOR CAN DO FOR YOU

12

Removing Moles,
Growths, Brown Spots,
and Discolorations

Facial skin is host to a wide variety of growths and color changes, some with long and complicated-sounding medical names. In general, as you age, more growths become apparent. Though most of these growths, spots, and discolorations are *benign* (noncancerous, not dangerous to your health), they can become quite troublesome cosmetically. Many people opt for cosmetic surgery when their spots and growths can no longer be hidden by makeup. Doctors used the term *lesion* to refer to any lumps, bumps, or discolorations that in any way cause concern or that differ from normal skin. This chapter discusses some of the more common cosmetic lesions and covers the various chemical and surgical procedures to treat them.

Unfortunately, some people don't do anything about their unsightly growths, spots, or skin stains simply because they are not aware that anything can be done about them. Others do not have them removed because of fears: of pain, of scarring, of turning something harmless into cancer, or of the expense. Another common reason for not having cosmetic surgery—and one that never ceases to amaze me—is simply because, way back when, family doctors advised them that "if it doesn't bother you, don't bother it." These same people usually tell me that for years they have unsuccessfully tried to cover their moles, "beauty marks," "warts," and "liver spots" with makeup, and were *still* unhappy! If you can identify with any one of the fears or hesitations about cosmetic surgery, this chapter will serve to enlighten you about the relative safety, ease, and inexpensiveness involved in making yourself look and feel better. Fortunately, many refinements in surgical techniques have occurred over the years, and many people can benefit esthetically and psychologically by cosmetic surgery.

In short, removing growths, spots, and discolorations generally causes little discomfort during or after the procedures, requires little or no loss of time from work, and needs minimal postsurgical care. In many cases, the surgical wounds may even be covered with makeup after just forty-eight hours.

In the following sections, I discuss the more common in-office cosmetic surgical procedures that are available for removing a variety of common facial skin problems, such as moles, warts, keratoses, cysts, overgrown oil glands, and skin tags. The pros and cons of each treatment will be discussed. Many of these same surgical procedures are also used for treating more serious, noncosmetic skin growths, such as precancers and cancers (see Chapter 17).

The following section, which is of a more general nature, is intended to give you sufficient information to intelligently appreciate what cosmetic in-office surgery is all about, so that you can better understand your doctor's specific recommendations. However, this information is not a substitute for a frank discussion between you and your doctor regarding what is best for you. Naturally, any questions or concerns you have about any procedure should be discussed with your doctor *before* you proceed with surgery. Afterwards may be too late.

TYPES OF ANESTHESIA

Local Anesthetics

Most in-office surgery is uncomfortable enough to necessitate the administration of a local anesthetic. The first question that people ask about almost any surgical procedure, no matter how minor, is: "Will it hurt?" For most procedures, the doctor injects a small amount of xylocaine (lidocaine) or procaine under the spot to be removed to numb the area. Xylocaine acts much like the novocaine dentists frequently use, except that lidocaine works almost instantly. The surgeon using lidocaine on the face does not need to wait twenty minutes for the painkilling effects to work. Usually by the time the needle is withdrawn, the area is already numb. A small, ultrathin needle is most frequently used. This needle is generally much finer than an ordinary sewing needle. As the needle enters your skin, you will feel a small pinprick. Most of my patients describe the discomfort of the anesthetic as equivalent to a mosquito bite. A few more sensitive patients claim that it feels more like a bee sting. What you will actually feel will depend upon your general threshold for pain and which area of your face is being anesthetized.

Following the injection, you will experience a slight burning sensation that will last from one to three seconds, after which the injected area will become numb. Anesthetics eliminate pain, but not the sensation of pressure. You may still be able to feel the doctor pressing on an anesthetized area while he or she works, but you will not feel pain.

If your doctor uses xylocaine combined with epinephrine (adrenaline), the anesthesia will usually last approximately sixty to ninety minutes. If not, the anesthesia will wear off in about thirty minutes.

Following most in-office surgical procedures, you will usually experience little discomfort after the anesthesia has worn off, though you may occasionally feel some throbbing or slight tenderness for a day or so. If for some reason your doctor anticipates that you may have more than the usual postsurgical discomfort, he or she may prescribe analgesics (painkillers).

Certain areas of your face are more sensitive to the injection of local anesthetic than others, such as the area around your mouth, especially the upper lip and around your nose. Your cheeks and temples are generally less so. Most of you would probably cringe at the thought of getting an injection near your eyes. Surprisingly, however, the eyelids are not particularly sensitive areas to locally anesthetize. The reason for these differences has something to do with the stretchability of skin.

The elasticity or inelasticity of a particular area of your skin plays a major role in determining how uncomfortable an injection of anesthetic is going to be. Whenever an anesthetic is administered, the injected fluid temporarily stretches the skin tissues of that area. The more inelastic the skin, the more uncomfortable an injection is likely to be. Stretching a relatively inelastic area, such as your upper lip, can be quite uncomfortable. On the other hand, precisely because eyelids are so stretchable, they are one of the least uncomfortable areas to anesthetize. Many people also harbor the fear that the needle is going to go directly through their lids into their eyes. In fact, the needle is placed very superficially into the eyelid skin, far from the eyeball itself.

Nitrous Oxide
("Sweet Air" or "Laughing Gas")

Many of you are probably familiar with *nitrous oxide* ("sweet air" or "laughing gas") from your visits to the dentist. The use of nitrous oxide gas can be an extremely effective means of calming patients and reducing operative pain. It is referred to as "conscious sedation," because you are not actually "put to sleep," but instead are put into a relaxed state of sedation.

Through a nasal mask, you inhale a mixture of nitrous oxide and oxygen gases, yet all the while you remain fully conscious and able to follow instructions. However, your sensitivity to discomfort is lessened. Many people experience a pleasant kind of high, as if they have had several drinks. After the surgical procedure is over, you breathe oxygen to clear out your lungs. In a few minutes, all the effects of the nitrous oxide are usually gone.

I personally find "sweet air" particularly useful for the squeamish, anxious, or needle-shy individual. I routinely use it in my office for performing a number of different surgical procedures. For pain control and sedation, nitrous oxide may be used alone, in combination with a local anesthetic, or just briefly to allow a local anesthetic to be more comfortably administered. Unfortunately, most dermatologists have not been trained in its use and it is, therefore, not widely available at this time.

You should not confuse nitrous oxide sedation with general anesthesia. When your doctor suggests giving you nitrous oxide gas, he or she is not talking about giving you general anesthesia and putting you out completely. They are also *not* referring to ether. This confusion with general anesthesia and/or ether has unfortunately prevented a number of people from taking advantage of sweet air when it was offered to them.

Skin Refrigerant Sprays

Topical anesthetic sprays, such as *ethyl chloride* or *flurethyl spray*, are two other anesthetics that your doctor may have occasion to use. These anesthetics are sometimes called *skin refrigerants* because they work by temporarily freezing the surface of your skin and briefly numbing the nerves. Their effects last only a few seconds, and their use is usually restricted to those surgical procedures that may be performed very quickly. They are also used to pre-numb an area so that a local anesthetic may be injected more comfortably.

COMMON COSMETIC SURGICAL METHODS

Shave Excision

Shave excision (removal) is an excellent method for removing growths elevated above the skin surface. Immediately following the administration of the anesthetic, the doctor uses a scalpel to remove the unwanted growth with a horizontal, back and forth, "sawing" motion of the scalpel blade (Figure 4a). Shave excision essentially consists of "sculpting" the unwanted growth away from the surrounding normal skin. The wound underneath is then left to heal by itself; no *sutures* ("stitches") are usually required. Since the wound that is created is very superficial, there is generally little risk of scarring with shave excisions. The cosmetic result is usually excellent.

Scissor Excision

Scissor excision or scissor removal is essentially a variation of shave excision, except that instead of a scalpel, a delicate surgical scissors is used to cut away the growth. Once again, no stitches are generally required and healing is usually quite cosmetically satisfying.

Excision

When doctors use the term *excision* by itself, they frequently mean that the unwanted tissue will be more deeply removed with a scalpel and that sutures will probably be required (Figures 4b, c). Typically, the surgeon cuts through several layers of skin. The skin is usually cut out in the shape of an ellipse; at the end, the wound is drawn into a fine line by stitches. Unfortunately, whenever skin is deeply cut, a small scar is likely to result.

To make any anticipated scar less obvious and more cosmetically acceptable, the plastic surgeon or dermatologic surgeon does several things. First, when performing an excision, the doctor carefully chooses the directions of his cuts so that the final scar will blend almost imperceptibly with the natural tension and wrinkle lines of the skin. In addition, to prevent stitch tracts (cross-hatched scarring), the surgeon uses ultrafine suture material on the face. And since stitch tracts are more likely to

FIGURE 4.

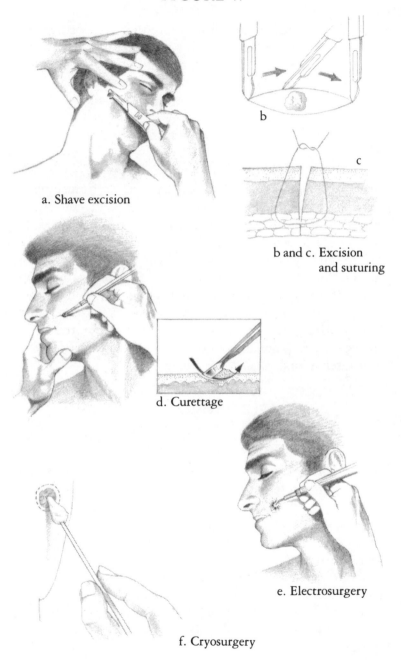

a. Shave excision

b

c

b and c. Excision
    and suturing

d. Curettage

e. Electrosurgery

f. Cryosurgery

occur when stitches are left in for more than four or five days, most doctors remove them on the third or fourth day after surgery. Once the stitches are removed, the wound is usually redressed with thin strips of tape (e.g., STERI-STRIPS, skin closure tapes), which are used in place of the stitches to hold the wound edges together until healing is complete.

Curettage

Curettage is a kind of surgical skin scraping performed with a special instrument called a *curet*, hence the name curettage. A curet is a cutting instrument with a round or oval, loop-shaped cutting edge and a handle, and is available in varying sizes (Figure 4d). Larger curets are used for removing larger growths. Curets are used to "scoop" out or off an unwanted growth. If the growths to be removed are small, your doctor may remove them without giving a prior anesthetic, since the process of anesthetizing in that case may be more uncomfortable than curettage itself. Wounds from curettage are usually left to heal by themselves and require no sutures.

ELECTROSURGERY

Electrodessication

Electrodessication is a technique where the dermatologist uses a high frequency, alternating electric current to dry up (*dehydrate*) unwanted growths. A fine probe through which the electric current passes is held in contact with the growth (Figure 4e). The growth is destroyed by small bursts of spark-producing electric current. A local anesthetic is usually required for treating large growths. For treating multiple small growths, many people prefer not to have anesthesia, claiming that the anesthetic injections are more uncomfortable than the procedure itself. Wounds are left to heal by themselves and do not require suturing.

Electrocoagulation
and Electrocautery

Both these electrosurgical methods rely upon the use of intense heat to destroy unwanted tissue. A treatment probe is placed in contact with the growth. When the electric current is applied, intense heat is generated and the unwanted tissue is literally "boiled" or, more technically put, *coagulated*. Electrocoagulation is usually reserved for destroying larger amounts of unwanted tissue, but because more tissue is destroyed the possibility of scar formation does exist. Wounds created by both electrocoagulation and electrocautery do not require suture closure and are left to heal by themselves.

CRYOSURGERY

Cryosurgery (*cryo* = cold) is simply the use of freezing to destroy unwanted tissue. *Liquid nitrogen* is currently the most frequently used of all freezing agents. Dry ice, a solid carbon dioxide, is also occasionally used. Liquid nitrogen freezes the unwanted growth and lowers its temperature to minus 195 degrees centigrade at its surface, and to between minus 70 and minus 125 degrees centigrade within it. Because of the numbing effect of the extreme cold, freezing is only slightly uncomfortable and no local anesthesia is generally required.

Liquid nitrogen is commonly applied either with a cotton-tipped (swab-like) applicator (Figure 4f), or by spraying it on. More than one application at each treatment session may be necessary. The amount of time that the liquid nitrogen must be kept in contact with the skin depends upon the size and depth of the unwanted growth to be treated. As a rule, larger lesions require longer contact time. In general, each application requires between fifteen and ninety seconds. The site is then left to thaw. Sometimes, in order to completely remove a large growth, a second application of liquid nitrogen, immediately after the first, may be needed.

Cryosurgery destroys unwanted tissue by causing destructive ice crystal formation within its cells. Cryosurgery is generally accompanied by a slight stinging or burning sensation. The discomfort peaks during thawing, about two minutes following treatment. Normally, within three to six hours after treatment, a blister forms at the treatment site. This blister dries up within two to three days and subsequently scales off in about three weeks. Freezing growths on the ears, eyelids, and around the lips is generally more uncomfortable than elsewhere on the face. No stitches or special bandages are required for wound healing. Cryosurgery with liquid nitrogen poses little risk of scarring. However, since the skin's pigment cells (melanocytes) are highly sensitive to extreme cold, loss of normal skin color in the treated area can occasionally occur.

DERMABRASION

Dermabrasion is a form of skin planing or skin sanding which is performed with rapidly rotating brushes. Before dermabrading the face, the skin is thoroughly frozen with a skin refrigerant spray, such as ethyl chloride or flurethyl spray. Dermabrasion has enjoyed its greatest success in the treatment of certain cases of extensive acne scarring. For that reason, I have chosen to leave the discussion of dermabrasion for Chapter 13, which deals with the various treatments for scarring.

HOW SURGICAL WOUNDS HEAL

If you are contemplating cosmetic surgery, you need to know something about how surgical wounds normally heal. It's a fact: wound sites right after surgery are not particularly attractive to look at. Learning that simple fact *after* your surgery, rather than before, can be quite distressing, not to mention the source of much immediate dissatisfaction with the outcome of the procedure.

It seems to be basic human nature to want and expect to see immediate cosmetic improvement as soon as the bandages are removed. Instead, people are often quite disappointed to see a swollen, healing wound. Fortunately, this disappointment lasts only a short time until wound healing and swelling have subsided. If you are aware of what to expect *beforehand*, you are less likely to be temporarily disappointed and unhappy with the immediate outcome of your cosmetic procedure.

Uncomplicated wound healing follows a regular progression. For about one to two weeks after surgery, the center of the wound will be raw and oozing. Within a few days, you will usually see an angry-looking reddish halo, looking something like the corona of the sun, fanning out from the center of the wound. You may think that the oozing and the reddish halo are signs of infection. They aren't. That's just normal healing. Of course, if you have any specific questions, you should call your doctor.

Most wounds form a crust or "scab" within the first one to two weeks following surgery. In turn, the crust usually falls off between the second and third week after surgery. At that point, the wound usually is a bright pink or reddish color. It's the same kind of color that you find after a scab on a scrape or cut falls off. During the next several weeks, the reddish color turns a dark brown and then proceeds to slowly fade to normal color. The wound progresses through a series of intermediate color changes; usually medium brown, light brown, and fawn-colored. All of these color changes are collectively referred to as *postinflammatory hyperpigmentation*. In plain talk, after any injury to your skin, you can expect your skin to become temporarily "stained" as part of the healing process. I'm sure you can imagine how upset some people feel when, for example, they've had a mole removed from their face and then find a dark brown spot in its place, but weren't told to expect it.

Postsurgical skin stains may take between six weeks and six

months to fade. In general, in light-skinned individuals, they fade sooner; in dark or black-skinned people, they take longer. You may safely use makeup to cover the discoloration during the waiting period. While patience and reassurance are needed to get through this often difficult waiting time, most people will quickly admit that it was well worth it.

LASERS

The word *laser* conjures up almost futuristic, *Star Wars*-like images in many people's minds. Increasingly, we read about the successful medical uses of lasers for removal of tattoos or special, disfiguring blood vessel overgrowths, called "port wine" stains. More recently, they are being tested in the treatment of an increasing number of skin growths, which will be discussed later in this chapter.

Laser machines and laser treatments remain expensive. So far, however, except for the treatment of certain blood vessel overgrowths, lasers have not demonstrated any significant benefits over the simpler, often far less costly techniques discussed earlier in this chapter. A more detailed discussion of what laser therapy is all about, and especially its role in the treatment of certain types of blood vessel overgrowths, will be found in Chapter 13.

COSMETIC CHEMOSURGERY

(Chemical Applications, Chemical Peels)

The application of caustic acids to remove brown spots and blotchy, irregular pigmentation of the skin has been used for over sixty years and is sometimes referred to as *cosmetic chemosurgery, chemical applications,* or *chemical peels.* While not strictly surgery, the use of acids for treating certain kinds of lesions is routinely used by many dermatologists and other cosmetic surgeons.

Nowadays, trichloroacetic acid (TCA), in varying strengths, and phenol are the two most commonly used acids. Depending upon the particular purpose or site for which it is intended, the strength of TCA for cosmetic chemosurgery can be varied. These acids superficially "burn away" the unwanted tissue. In the next chapter, I describe more fully the specific methods involved in extensive chemical peeling to "freshen" facial skin and to treat wrinkles. In this chapter, my focus is the chemical applications for treating small brown spots, color irregularities, and certain other kinds of benign skin lesions.

Here's what you can expect with a chemical application. Following cleaning and degreasing of your skin with alcohol or acetone, either phenol or TCA is applied directly to the unwanted spot. Within fifteen to thirty seconds you will begin to feel a strong burning sensation and, within one to two minutes, the treated area will turn a chalk white. At that point, your doctor neutralizes the acid with water or alcohol, stopping the burning. Within a half hour, redness and swelling begin, and the chalk white area usually turns a burnt-orange or onion skin-like hue. During the course of the next two weeks, the treated area will slough and scale off and along with it goes the unwanted growth or discoloration.

As a rule, you will experience some mild discomfort after the procedure, but it usually doesn't last for more than twenty-four to forty-eight hours. In most cases, I permit makeup to be worn forty-eight hours after treatment. Since postinflammatory staining of your skin can be pronounced after chemical applications, I feel that the early use of makeup can be psychologically uplifting during the often anxious healing period. However, a few people must wait seven to twelve days before applying makeup.

You must avoid overexposure to the sun after chemical applications. In general, sun exposure should be restricted for the first two to three months after treatment. For this reason, I usually perform chemical applications in the late autumn or early winter, before the sunny season gets under way. If for some reason you must travel to sunny areas, sunscreens should be diligently applied at all times. Permanent dark patches sometimes occur following excessive sun exposure, particularly within the first two months after chemical applications.

However, usually few complications occur, especially when only a few or small areas are treated by chemical application. The main advantages of limited chemical applications are that they may be performed quickly and require no local anesthesia or cutting of the skin. Results are generally quite satisfactory.

COMMON BENIGN
LESIONS AND
THEIR TREATMENTS

The following sections cover the most common types of facial skin growths and discolorations, as well as the various alternatives for treating them. As before, the pros and cons of each of the alternatives are discussed.

Moles

A mole, or "beauty mark" or "birthmark," as it is called by many people, or *nevus* (plural: nevi), as your dermatologist might call it, is simply a benign overgrowth of pigment cells. Moles may be flesh-colored or, more frequently, may vary in color from light to dark browns. They may be flat or raised, have broad bases or grow on stalks, and can range in size from a pinhead to several inches long. Depending upon their size, shape, and location, moles may be removed by shave, scissor, or deep excision methods. Although frequently performed by many surgeons and plastic surgeons, I seldom recommend deep excision of a mole.

While electrosurgery, cryosurgery, or chemosurgery may give comparable cosmetic results, they should not be performed on moles because these methods destroy tissue beyond recognition. They make it impossible for a skin pathologist to examine the mole under the microscope.

It is important to realize that though you may be opting for cosmetic surgery only, the removed growth will most likely be *biopsied*, or removed and sent for microscopic examination, rather than thrown out in the surgical wastebin. This is done because, on occasion, benign-appearing growths, which were removed for cosmetic reasons only, were found to have evidence of malignant changes in them. Obviously, fortuitous discoveries like that can sometimes prove lifesaving.

I prefer shave excision for removing most moles, especially those which protrude above the skin surface. With shave excision, the mole can be "sculpted" away from the underlying and surrounding skin, while preserving the general contours of the region. Because shave excision removes only the surface of the mole, leaving the below-surface remainder in place, regrowth or darkening of the treatment site occasionally occurs sometime in the future. However, this occurs infrequently, and if it does, the treatment area can easily be touched-up with light electrosurgery in a matter of minutes. Those surgeons who favor deep excision of moles point out that recurrences seldom occur because even the deepest portion of the mole is removed. Nevertheless, I feel that deep excision requires the placement of stitches and poses the risk of leaving you with a permanent linear scar and stitch marks.

Seborrheic Keratoses
(Senile Keratoses,
"Heaped-up Age Spots")

Seborrheic keratoses are the most common skin growths occurring in middle to later life. There is often a strong family history for their development. Many people frequently mistake seborrheic keratoses for warts. They aren't warts, though certain types can closely resemble them. In my practice, I often refer to them simply as "heaped-up, passage-of-time" spots.

Seborrheic keratoses are benign, pigmented overgrowths of skin. They are typically thick, "stuck-on," scaly, greasy-looking masses that may be found in shades of yellow or, more commonly, faint to extremely dark brown. Since they are quite superficially located in the skin, simple curettage is the most effective method for removing them.

Seborrheic keratoses may be removed by electrosurgery, cryosurgery, or deep excision, although I don't ordinarily use any of these methods. Cryosurgery poses a risk of loss of normal skin color in the treated area. Owing to the possibility of damage to the underlying skin by the electric current or heat, electrosurgery poses a small risk of scarring. In my opinion, deep excision of a seborrheic keratosis should never be performed, since their superficial location in the skin does not justify deeper cutting.

Viral Growths— ### Warts and Molluscum

Two types of benign viral growths commonly affect the skin: common warts (*veruccae*), and a less well-known, but often equally troublesome problem with an imposing name, *molluscum contagiosum*. Besides being cosmetically embarrassing, there is another compelling reason you should seek medical attention for these conditions. Since both warts and molluscum are caused by viruses, both are potentially contagious, or *spreadable,* not only to other areas of your own skin, but to other people.

Three varieties of true warts can affect your face: common warts, filiform warts, and flat warts. All are caused by types of wart viruses called *human papillomaviruses.* Common warts appear as flesh-colored, rugged-surfaced bumps, and tiny pinpoint, black specks may stipple their surface. Filiform warts are soft, slender, fingerlike growths. Flat warts are flesh-colored or tan, soft, flat-topped bumps.

For treating numerous flat warts of the face, I recommend the use of electrosurgery. For common warts, I usually use electrosurgery followed by curettage. For filiform warts, I prefer scissor excision followed by electrosurgery of the wound base. Cryosurgery is an excellent alternative method for treating warts. Because of their superficial location in the skin, scalpel excision is unwarranted for the removal of any type of wart.

Prescription or nonprescription antiwart acid preparations are also sometimes recommended for home use, especially for treating multiple warts or for use between surgical treatments. These wart therapies may occasionally be successful, but it normally takes several weeks of daily applications to achieve success. Most people find home therapy a nuisance and often forget to follow the regimen that their doctor has outlined for them.

Molluscum contagiosum lesions are flesh-colored, waxy-looking bumps that are elevated above the surface and have a central depression right on their peaks. They are shaped something like burned-out volcanoes. If you see one, look more carefully. You will often find others nearby.

While I prefer simple curettage for removing molluscum, equally satisfactory results can be obtained with liquid nitrogen cryotherapy or electrosurgery. Excision is not warranted because molluscum lesions are not deep. Chemical application of TCA is sometimes also used to treat them, although repeated applications are frequently necessary. Home use, antiwart and acid therapies, such as those already described, may also sometimes be helpful, although the same reservations about their effectiveness apply here.

Solar Lentigines
("Age Spots," "Liver Spots")

Solar lentigines, which usually appear later in life, hence the name age spots, are light or dark brown and generally appear against the backdrop of heavily sundamaged or weather-beaten skin. They usually range in size from a quarter of an inch to one to two inches in diameter.

Superficial electrosurgery, cryosurgery, and chemical application give comparably satisfactory cosmetic results. Nevertheless, I prefer light electrosurgery for treating solar lentigines. After electrosurgery, the brown spots can literally be wiped away with a gauze sponge. I find that there is more chance of prolonged postinflammatory skin staining with liquid nitrogen cryotherapy, or TCA, or phenol chemical applications. Furthermore, after electrosurgery, you need not hide from the sun as you must do after chemical applications.

Solar lentigines should not be confused with freckles (*ephelides*). Freckles are very common small brown spots that appear in childhood, especially on sun-exposed areas. They tend to fade in adulthood, but can become darker and more obvious with sun overexposure. Usually when sunlight is avoided and appropriate sunscreens are used freckles do not cause much cosmetic concern. When they are more numerous and cosmetically troublesome, they can be treated with chemical peels or dermabrasion (Chapter 13).

Xanthelasmas
(Fatty Eyelid Deposits)

Xanthelasmas are raised, soft, yellowish deposits of cholesterol and fat not uncommonly found on the lower and, more frequently, upper eyelids. About 25 percent of those people who have them are found to have elevated blood cholesterol levels. For this reason, before focusing on the cosmetic aspects of xanthelasmas, I send all my patients who have them for a blood test to check their cholesterol level.

Xanthelasmas may be effectively removed by chemical application of trichloroacetic acid, electrosurgery, cryosurgery, excision, or scissor excision. The cosmetic results after any of these methods are usually excellent. Large, thicker xanthelasmas treated by chemical application often require several treatment sessions to achieve the desired results.

Sebaceous Gland Hyperplasia
("Overgrown Oil Glands")

Oil gland overgrowths are usually round and lobed-surfaced, ivory or yellowish, waxy-looking bumps. They are commonly found on the faces of middle-aged to elderly people. Usually several are present. It is unusual to have just one.

Electrosurgery to flatten these growths until they are flush with the surrounding skin surface works quite well. However, since these growths extend quite deeply below the surface, the flattened spot that remains after electrosurgery frequently appears waxy-yellow. Unfortunately, the flattened oil glands do tend, after some time, to regrow and require retreatment. At the same time, new ones may continue to form elsewhere. Cryosurgery has also been found helpful in certain cases. However, at best, the cosmetic results would be no better than with electrosurgery, and the risk of skin color loss, as always, must be considered. Excision surgery would completely remove the growth, but it is not advisable because of the possibility of trading a sebaceous gland overgrowth for a line scar and stitch tracks.

Milia (Tiny Sebaceous Cysts)

Milia are small sebaceous cysts that closely resemble whiteheads. While occasionally only one or two milia are seen, most often many can be found. When there are few, your doctor may just nick the top of them with a fine scalpel or needle and express the contents. If they are numerous, electrosurgery is preferable and cosmetically quite satisfactory.

Using electrosurgery, the dermatologist can remove even hundreds of milia in a matter of minutes. If you have numerous milia, it becomes too impractical and uncomfortable to locally anesthetize all treatment sites. In this case, the use of sweet air (nitrous oxide) sedation can be useful, particularly if you have a low pain tolerance. Following electrosurgery, tiny crusts form. These fall off within about five to seven days, leaving a tiny reddish spot. The redness usually fades during the next two weeks.

Acrochordons
(Skin Tags, Papillomas)

Skin tags are small, flesh-colored benign growths that usually hang on fine stalks. They are frequently found on the sides of the neck and the eyelids, as well as other areas of the body. Skin tags may also appear from light to dark brown in color. There is usually a strong family history for developing them.

Scissor excision, cryosurgery, and electrosurgery can all be successfully used to remove skin tags. For multiple small skin tags, I prefer to use electrocautery. The small, charred crusts usually fall off in five to seven days and complete healing occurs over the next two weeks. For larger growths, I prefer scissor excision followed by electrocautery of the base of the wound. The cosmetic results of both these methods are usually excellent. While treated lesions do not usually recur, *new* skin tags do tend to appear with time. Removal procedures often have to be repeated every one to five years. While cryosurgery also works well, I don't feel the risk of possible pigment loss at the treatment sites is worth using it.

13

Eliminating Wrinkles,
Scars, and
"Broken" Blood Vessels

While no fountain of youth has yet been found, medical science has and is hard at work developing new methods to improve our appearance and make our skin look as though the hands of time had been pushed back.

Where once expensive and often uncomfortable surgical procedures, such as face-lifts and dermabrasions, requiring long recuperation periods and lost time from work, were the only medical means for dealing with wrinkles and scars, science has now reduced the need for these procedures through the near-"magic" of a simple injection. A few years ago, injectable silicone was the only thing available for wrinkle removal, and even it could be obtained from only a handful of dermatologists around the country. More recently, however, injectable collagen has become widely available for many of the same cosmetic purposes. Both silicone and collagen are used to plump up and smooth out wrinkle lines and skin creases and to fill in depressed scars.

INJECTABLES FOR
ELIMINATING WRINKLES
AND SCARS

Silicone (dimethyl siloxane) injections for the correction of wrinkles and depressed scars have been used for approximately thirty years. For most of those years, it was the only injectable substance available for these purposes, yet it was never granted Food and Drug Administration approval. Today, medical-grade silicones are still being used by a few practitioners for the treatment of wrinkles and depressed acne scars, and these physicians claim to obtain cosmetically satisfactory results with their patients.

Silicone is an inert, non-organic substance which is injected into the skin in a liquid form. It is generally injected very slowly, droplet by droplet, and each drop is massaged gently to spread the liquid evenly through the tissue. There is a slight disruption of the tissue underneath the skin when the silicone droplets are dispersed, causing a local collection of collagen and cells around each droplet of silicone. The plumping out and elimination of the overlying wrinkles or depressed scars result from a combination of the silicone droplets themselves and the collection of surrounding tissue material. Silicone is not biodegradable. Once injected into the skin, it remains there, permanent and unchanged; therefore, touch-up injections are rarely necessary.

However, there are drawbacks. Silicone droplets are extremely difficult and often impossible to remove once they have been injected. Moreover, the droplets have been known to shift from their original locations in the skin, especially in cases where the silicone liquid was improperly injected. This shifting has resulted in the formation of odd-looking bumps at sites distant from the original injection. These bumps may be either flesh-colored, if noninflamed, or pinkish, if inflamed. Treatment of these bumps has, in some cases, involved injection of an anti-inflammatory substance, and in others, surgical removal.

Since silicone is not biodegradable and cannot be removed, the question of the shifting droplets has been the source of much heated controversy between silicone's supporters and detractors, and has contributed greatly to silicone's lack of widespread popularity through the years.

Supporters of silicone claim that any previously reported problems with it stem from use by inexperienced physicians, use of too much silicone at each treatment site, and use of less pure (nonmedical grade), adulterated forms of silicone. Nevertheless, since the advent of FDA-approved injectable collagen (ZYDERM collagen) for the treatment of wrinkles and acne scarring, I no longer recommend silicone injections for my patients.

Injectable collagen or ZYDERM collagen is a highly purified form of collagen made from calf skin. Collagen is a natural structural protein found in all parts of your body. After six years of extensive testing, injectable collagen was given FDA approval in 1981 for cosmetic use in the treatment of smile and *frown lines* (Figure 5a), acne, and postsurgical depressed scars. Since that time ZYDERM collagen has been used in more than two hundred fifty thousand patients.

The collagen in ZYDERM collagen should not be confused with the collagen found in many popular moisturizing creams and lotions. As I emphasized in Chapter 2, the collagen protein molecule is too large to be "eaten" up by your skin from a moisturizer. However, ZYDERM collagen, by being *injected*, is placed by your doctor right where it is needed. To be successful, treatment sites must be overcorrected, that is, your doctor must inject enough collagen into each treatment site to elevate that area *twice as high as it was originally deep*. This explains the mosquito bite-like bump found at the injection site right after an injection. Within twenty-four to seventy-two hours, the overcorrection disappears, as the salt water in which the ZYDERM collagen is suspended is reabsorbed by your body.

Immediately following treatment, the injection sites will look pinkish or bruised, and slightly swollen. The desired cosmetic improvement becomes apparent once the treatment sites return to normal, within one to three days. You may even return to work immediately after a treatment session. If you wish to keep the treatment a secret, the bumps may be explained away as a case of hives. The total number of injections, and the amount of collagen needed, depend upon the location and

FIGURE 5. *Methods of wrinkle and scar removal*

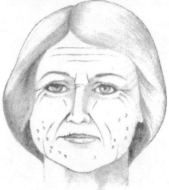

"Ice-pick" scar

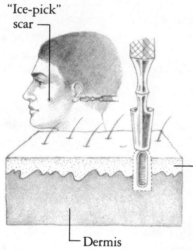

a. Wrinkles and scars treatable by Zyderm

Epidermis

b. Punch-graft. Skin from behind the ear is grafted into an "ice pick" acne scar.

Dermis

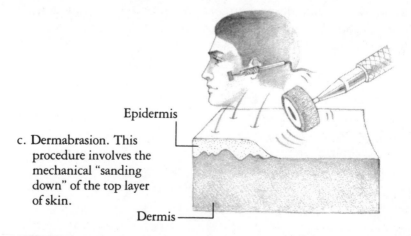

Epidermis

c. Dermabrasion. This procedure involves the mechanical "sanding down" of the top layer of skin.

Dermis

severity of the scars or wrinkles being treated. The deeper the wrinkle or scar, or the more tightly bound the fibrous tissue of the scar below the skin surface, the more collagen will be required to elevate it.

Treatment sessions are usually spaced at two- to four-week intervals. In general, depending upon the specific condition being treated, cosmetic improvement may be observed after two to six treatment sessions. The same natural forces, such as smiling, laughing, eating, sun exposure, etc., that originally wore down your native collagen and led to wrinkling in the first place, continue despite ZYDERM collagen therapy, and even go to work on ZYDERM collagen. Therefore, touch-up ZYDERM collagen injections are needed periodically to maintain the correction.

ZYDERM collagen does not correct all acne scarring or wrinkling equally well. As a rule, shallow, depressed, pock mark scars respond quite well to ZYDERM collagen. Similarly, frown lines on the sides of the nose and mouth, the deep grooves at the corners of the mouth and between the eyes respond quite well to collagen injections. On the other hand, deeply pitted, so-called "ice-pick" scars do not generally respond well to injectable collagen. The horizontal furrow lines of the forehead also tend to respond less dramatically. In addition, chicken-pox scars, because they are very tightly bound to the underlying tissue, do not respond well to ZYDERM collagen. For people with these problems, other corrective cosmetic surgical procedures, which are discussed later in this chapter, are recommended.

Two types of ZYDERM collagen are currently available: ZYDERM collagen I and ZYDERM collagen II. ZYDERM collagen I contains approximately one-half the concentration of collagen contained in ZYDERM collagen II (35 percent vs. 65 percent collagen). The remainder is simple physiologic salt water (*saline*). At the present time, ZYDERM collagen I is favored by most cosmetic surgeons for treating the majority of scar and wrinkle problems. Where the scars or furrows are exceptionally deep, however, ZYDERM collagen II has been found to be quite beneficial.

A few people have experienced bumps following treatment with either form of ZYDERM collagen. Sometimes these bumps have persisted at the treatment sites for several weeks or occasionally have appeared at previous treatment sites after periods of intense sun exposure, vigorous exercise, or heavy alcohol consumption. However, such reactions are infrequent, generally short-lived, and resolve by themselves. The problem of persistent bumpiness after injections is somewhat more common with ZYDERM collagen II. Because of this, a skin defect is usually treated with ZYDERM collagen II to the point of correction, rather than overcorrection, as it is with ZYDERM collagen I.

Unfortunately, not everyone is a suitable candidate for ZYDERM collagen therapy. Individuals with personal histories of *autoimmune diseases* (immunologic disorders), such as *lupus erythematosus, polyarteritis, polymyositis, rheumatoid* and *psoriatic arthritis* should not be treated with injectable collagen. Everyone else is screened with a skin test given four weeks before actual treatments are to start.

A ZYDERM collagen skin test is performed to insure that a particular candidate is not sensitive to the injectable collagen formulation. A small amount of test material is injected into the forearm. Approximately 96 percent get the green light. About 3 percent of individuals given the test dose will be found sensitive to collagen and will not be candidates for treatment. Another 1 percent will develop sensitivity to collagen after treatments have begun and, unfortunately, will no longer be able to receive collagen injections.

In my opinion, the introduction of injectable ZYDERM collagen for the cosmetic treatment of wrinkles and depressed scars overall has been a significant step forward in cosmetic surgery. A newer form of injectable collagen for the treatment of deeper defects, and a noncollagen injectable for the treatment of wrinkles and scars currently under investigation, are discussed in Chapter 18.

COSMETIC SURGERY
FOR PITTED
("ICE-PICK") SCARS

Ice-pick scars are narrow, deeply pitted, tightly bound down scars with rigid walls resulting from severe acne vulgaris. Three surgical methods are currently used to remove these scars: *punch-excision, punch-elevation,* and *punch-grafting* (Figure 5b).

Chickenpox scars are occasionally treated by these same methods. Each is an in-office procedure that can be performed in just a few minutes under local anesthesia.

Punch-Excision

Following the administration of local anesthesia beneath the scar, a cookie-cutter-like instrument called a *punch* is used to remove a plug of scar tissue. Punches come in varying sizes to fit the sizes of scars that are treated. The plug of tissue taken out is slightly wider than the pit scar to ensure that the entire scar is removed. The plug of scar is discarded and the edges of the wound are then stitched together with a fine or ultrafine suture material. The stitches are taken out in three days and are replaced with STERI-STRIPS skin closure tapes until complete wound healing takes place.

Punch-Elevation

Once again, following the administration of local anesthesia, a plug of pitted scar tissue is punched out. The plug of scar tissue, however, rather than being discarded, is instead elevated and positioned slightly above the level of the surrounding skin. The elevated plug is held in place by a STERI-STRIP tape until healing occurs. Once healing is complete, electrosurgery can be used both to flatten the elevated plug until it is level with the surrounding skin, and to "freshen up" its surface.

Punch-Grafting

As with punch-excision, in *punch-grafting* the scar is punched out and discarded. However, instead of simply stitching the wound closed, it is filled in with a snugly fitting punch-graft taken from a locally anesthetized site (*donor site*) behind the ear. The skin from behind the ear matches the color and texture of facial skin at the *recipient site*. The graft is then stitched in place or anchored by STERI-STRIPS tape until healing is complete. Here again, electrosurgery subsequently may be needed to level and smooth the graft sites.

In many cases, even after the wounds have fully healed, a faint circular rim may be visible upon very close inspection around each graft site. At normal distances, these circular rims generally blend with the multitude of skin surface irregularities and discolorations that most people normally have. The rims are barely noticeable, unless purposefully brought to another person's attention.

CHEMICAL PEELS

In the last chapter, I discussed the use of chemical applications for the treatment of localized skin discolorations and certain types of growths. More extensive chemical peels, involving larger areas of the face, or the entire face, are successfully used to treat a variety of cosmetic problems, such as fine, cross-hatched wrinkles, sun-damaged skin, and shallower types of acne scarring. Chemical peels can "freshen" and make more radiant skin that is otherwise dull-looking. Wrinkles around the mouth (*rhytides*) and eyes ("*crow's feet*") respond particularly well to chemical peels. Chemical peels are not effective, however, for treating redundant, hanging skin folds, or jowls.

As with more localized forms of chemical applications, the two most commonly used caustic agents for chemical peels are phenol and trichloracetic acid, either alone or in combination.

These acids destroy the surface proteins of the skin with which they come into contact. The effect is like that of a second-degree burn. After the peel, the treated skin sloughs off and new skin regenerates. The underlying tissue usually becomes thicker and somewhat more wrinkle-resistant than before. The beneficial results of chemical peels may last for several years.

Not everyone is a candidate for chemical peeling. In general, fair-complected people respond better to chemical peels than do dark-complected people, largely because they exhibit less color contrast between treated and untreated skin. Individuals with thick and oily skin also do not respond that well.

Full-face chemical peels basically differ little from localized chemical applications, except for the extent. The acids are applied with either cotton-tipped applicators or brushes. Usually one area of the face is treated at a time. Some physicians prefer to do one area of the face per treatment session.

When deep wrinkles are present, deeper peels are usually needed. In this case, the dermatologist may either apply more medication to each area or place an adhesive tape mask over the treated areas to "lock" in the chemicals. The tape mask is usually left on for twenty-four hours. Afterward, the healing process follows the same pattern that was described for localized chemical applications in Chapter 12.

Of course, since a larger area is being treated, somewhat more operative and postoperative discomfort is to be expected. This is easily managed by the administration of a tranquilizer before the procedure and a mild analgesic (pain pill) afterward. Postoperative discomfort rarely lasts longer than twenty-four to seventy-two hours. Excessive sun exposure must be avoided for at least two months following the chemical peel to minimize the chance of developing blotchy pigmentation. Makeup may be applied as soon as the crusts fall off.

In general, there are few complications with chemical peels. Occasionally, as I have mentioned, blotchy over- or under-pigmentation may occur. Rarely do *hypertrophic scars* ("proud flesh") develop. Should that occur, however, the scars may be treated by certain types of injections, which I describe later in this chapter.

DERMABRASION
(SKIN PLANING,
SKIN SANDING)

Dermabrasion has been used for well over thirty years for the treatment of scars and wrinkles. Its most frequent use has been for the improvement of acne scarring. It has also been successfully used to minimize chickenpox scars, keloids, and post-surgical scars. "Ice-pick" scars do not respond as satisfactorily as broader, more shallow, craterlike acne scars. By planing down the surrounding skin, acne craters become shallower and less noticeable. Here again, fair-complected individuals usually do better than dark-complected people.

Your doctor may perform dermabrasion using one or a combination of three basic types of dermabrading cutting tools: diamond fraises, wire brushes, and serrated wheels (Figure 5C). These cutting tools are attached to a rapidly rotating electric drill. Wire brushes are used for deeper cutting, and diamond fraises for more superficial planing. By varying the pressure with which they are applied, serrated wheels provide some of the advantages of both the diamond fraise and the wire brush.

Following local anesthesia, the facial skin is frozen solid with a skin refrigerant, such as ethyl chloride. Freezing enhances the anesthetic effect, but more importantly it stiffens the skin and makes a firm surface for dermabrasion. One area of the skin at a time is frozen and then treated.

Dermabrasion causes little operative discomfort, but is a somewhat messy procedure. The sanding causes a fine, mistlike spray of blood and skin. As a result, the doctor usually wears a welder's mask and the patient wears goggles. Following the procedure the entire face is bandaged.

For the first night, the patient is advised to sleep sitting up in order to reduce facial swelling. Painkillers are prescribed as needed. Alcohol consumption should be avoided. Antibacterial antibiotics and antiherpes simplex medications are prescribed to reduce the chances of infection. Crusts start to develop within a few days.

Shedding of the crusts begins by the end of the first week and is completed at the end of three weeks. Nevertheless, after ten days one is usually able to return to work. With this in mind, many dermabrasions are scheduled on Thursdays so that a patient can have two full weekends to recover and still be able to return to work on a Monday. Overexposure to sun must be avoided for at least three months after dermabrasion to avoid the development of blotchy pigmentation, particularly over-pigmentation. Postdermabrasion raised scars rarely develop. If they should, they can be treated by injections.

For properly selected candidates, dermabrasion can be a useful surgical method for treating wrinkles and scars. It can also be used to enhance the results of more extensive plastic surgical procedures, such as face-lifts.

TREATMENT OF
RAISED SCARS

There are basically two kinds of raised scars: *Hypertrophic* ("proud flesh") *scars* and *keloids*. Both types of scars may follow injury or surgery to the skin. At times, hypertrophic scars and keloids may look quite similar.

Very firm and pinkish in color, hypertrophic scars are essentially complications of wound healing. Instead of the normal healing that takes place at the site of a wound, the wound healing process seems to "overshoot" the mark, producing excess healing tissue that sticks up above the surrounding skin; hence the name "proud flesh." Frequently, hypertrophic scars will spontaneously flatten out in about six to nine months.

Keloids, which are very firm, flesh- to ivory-colored raised scars, can be quite similar in outward appearance to hypertrophic scars. However, keloids tend to grow to sizes well beyond the limits of the original wound sites.

Keloids can be rather cosmetically disfiguring. They may hang as large, pendulous growths from the earlobes, when they result from earpiercing. In general, black people are more prone to the formation of keloids, although Caucasians are by no means exempt. A familial predisposition exists for the development of keloids. If you are aware of such a tendency in your family you should tell your doctor about it *before* you undertake any cosmetic surgical procedures.

Hypertrophic scars are usually treated by a tincture of time. In other words, doctors usually allow a trial of several months to see whether they flatten out on their own. If not, a corticosteroid anti-inflammatory solution is injected directly into the scars to shrink them. These injections are referred to as *intralesional* or *therapeutic injections*. Intralesional injections for scars can be quite uncomfortable, since the doctor must exert significant pressure in order to force the medicine to evenly penetrate throughout the thick scar tissue. Several treatment sessions, spaced at two- to four-week intervals, are usually required to flatten a hypertrophic scar. Successful therapy results in a flat, ivory-colored spot that can be easily covered with makeup.

Keloids likewise can be shrunk significantly by intralesional steroid injections. However, the tendency of keloids to regrow often makes them more difficult to treat than hypertrophic scars. Surgical excision, followed by intralesional corticosteroid injections, and the application of surgical pressure dressings, are sometimes necessary to treat particularly resistant keloids.

Sometimes the dermatologist may try softening a keloid before injecting it by freezing it with liquid nitrogen and then allowing it to thaw. While freezing may make the injections less uncomfortable and more effective, there is a substantial risk that the treated area will permanently lose its normal color. For this reason, I seldom resort to this technique.

REMOVING "BROKEN" BLOOD VESSELS

Several different kinds of blood vessel problems may affect the face, giving it a streaked, blotchy, or ruddy look. Many people commonly refer to all of these blood vessel problems as "broken" blood vessels. Actually, in none of these conditions are the blood vessels really broken. In most cases, the "broken" blood vessels are really tiny, dilated blood vessels (capillaries) called *telangiectasias*. Sometimes the blood vessel that is dilated is a tiny artery called an *arteriole*. Because of the many "arms and legs" that seem to radiate from these dilated arterioles, these types of blood vessel problems are commonly referred to by doctors as "spider" hemangiomas, "spider" nevi, or "spider" telangiectasias.

Unfortunately, blood vessel blotching of the skin seldom disappears on their own. More often, the condition is permanent and, in fact, new blood vessels continue to appear with age. It is important for you to realize that all of these blood vessels are entirely superfluous. They serve no useful functions. They do not supply either nutrition or oxygen to your skin. The blood vessels deeper in your skin are responsible for those functions. All these abnormal blood vessel problems do is cause you needless cosmetic embarrassment.

While the exact causes for the development of telangiectasias and "spider" nevi are not known, several factors seem to aggravate these conditions. Alcohol, which ordinarily can dilate blood vessels, can aggravate the problem. In fact, the association between heavy alcohol intake and a flushed face with many dilated blood vessels is so well known that many people with facial blood vessel conditions come for treatment simply because they are tired of trying to convince others that they don't drink heavily.

"Broken" blood vessels are commonly found on badly sun-damaged skin. They can appear during pregnancy, although they generally disappear several weeks after delivery. They may be caused or worsened by constant exposure to excessive warmth. For this reason, many professional chefs have them.

People who tend to be *"flushers"* frequently develop numerous dilated blood vessels on their faces. "Flushers" are individuals who have a lifelong history of flushing easily and deeply when under emotional or physical stress, or simply after eating hot or very spicy foods. After years of dilating and constricting, the facial blood vessels of "flushers" lose some of their ability to constrict, and remain dilated and obvious.

Finally, people with certain underlying medical conditions, such as cirrhosis of the liver, scleroderma (a fibrosing connective tissue disease affecting the skin and other organs), and uncontrolled high blood pressure may also be troubled by the presence of numerous telangiectasias or "spiders." Of course, in these particular cases, attention should first be directed to remedying the underlying medical condition before attending to the cosmetic problem.

Electrodessication is the preferred method for eliminating telangiectasias and "spider" nevi. A fine epilating needle, like the type used for electrolysis of hairs, is inserted into a branching area of a telangiectasia or right into the central portion of the "spider" blood vessel. A small amount of electric current is delivered to the unwanted blood vessels, permanently closing them off and denying circulation to the radiating blood vessels. You may experience a momentary burning, stinging, or spark-like sensation as the electric current is delivered. Usually, as a reflex response (*not* from pain), your eyes may begin to water. No anesthesia is usually necessary and, in fact, local anesthesia can hinder the dermatologist by obscuring some of the finer blood vessels after it is injected. If you have a low pain threshold, nitrous oxide may be used.

Since your body is not "aware" of the useless nature of your "broken" blood vessels, your skin will often "try" to reform or rechannelize (the medical term is *recanalize*) the treated blood vessels after the treatment as part of its normal reparative functions. Because of this, one or more additional treatment sessions are usually needed to suppress any rechannelization.

Electrodessication has an excellent track record for eliminating unwanted facial blood vessels, even in those individuals who have a dense, "fishnet-like" arrangement of their telangiectasias. The main complication of electrodessication is the occasional formation of a dimple-like, tiny pit scar at the needle placement site. In general, pit scars rarely occur if the electric current is kept to the barest minimum to do the job.

PORT WINE STAINS
(NEVUS FLAMMAEUS)

The *port wine stain*, or *nevus flammaeus*, is another type of cosmetically troublesome blood vessel abnormality. Port wine stains are birthmarks composed of tiny, bunched-up blood vessels referred to by doctors as a *hemangiomas*. They are the most common of all vascular (blood vessel) birthmarks, and fortunately are most frequently found on the back of the scalp, well-hidden from view. However, they may affect any area of the body, even the mucous membranes of the mouth and nose. Although not hereditary, hemangiomas are somehow acquired during fetal development in the womb and are often present at birth. While port wine stains pose little serious threat to health, they can pose a serious cosmetic problem on an obvious area of the face.

Port wine stains are most often level with the surface of the surrounding skin and are some shade of red. They range from dime-sized to an area covering more than half the face. In time, some port wine stains turn deep red, reddish purple, or purplish, and may also develop colored lumps and bumps that can become quite prominent.

No therapy currently available can *entirely* eliminate port wine stains. Cryosurgery and dermabrasion have been tried, but scarring frequently occurs with their use, and they are generally no longer recommended for treating nevus flammaeus.

Tattooing

For flatter kinds of port wine stains, tattooing is sometimes used. Nontoxic skin pigments are tattooed into the port wine stain to lighten it up; however, it is usually impossible to completely mask. For lumpier hemangiomas, tattooing produces an even less acceptable cosmetic result. Furthermore, since the flesh-tinted tattooed areas cannot tan, they contrast sharply with tanned skin, making for a mottled appearance.

Lasers

The word *laser* is an acronym for *L*ight *A*mplification by *S*timulated *E*mission of *R*adiation. Simply stated, lasers are the focused beams of certain selected wavelengths of visible light. Three types are currently being used: the argon laser, the carbon dioxide laster, and the neodymium-YAG laser. At present, the most well-tested and most successful use of lasers has been in the treatment of port wine stains with the argon laser. Because they can provide substantial cosmetic improvement in certain cases where no therapy previously proved satisfactory, lasers represent a significant and exciting therapeutic advance in the treatment of port wine stains.

Hemoglobin, the red pigment of your red blood cells, highly and selectively absorbs the light from the argon laser. Directed to the hemoglobin pigment, the light from the argon laser passes straight through the skin and acts only within the blood vessels of the hemangioma where the hemoglobin pigment is concentrated. In general, therapy for port wine stains is more successful in adult patients who have widely dilated blood vessels. Successful therapy results in blanching of the treated areas. Even when complete blanching is not obtained, significant lightening in color is frequently possible. In general, port wine stains on the cheeks and neck respond better than those on the lips and chin. For large areas, laser therapy may require a year or more in order to achieve the desired results.

But laser therapy is not without its risks. Scarring and loss of color in the treatment areas can sometimes occur. To minimize this possibility, a small, one-half-inch test site in an out-of-the-way area (e.g., behind the ear, on the neck, or under the hairline) is selected for treatment. If no scarring or other adverse reactions occurs in the test area during the next three months, actual treatment of the entire lesion may be started.

In the properly selected patient, the results of argon laser therapy may be quite gratifying. Complete clearing is rare, but flattening and blanching of a port wine stain allow the person with this problem to apply masking cosmetics more easily and effectively (Chapter 4). At the present time, because there is much less experience using the other kinds of lasers, I have chosen to reserve discussion of them for Chapter 18.

TOPICAL RETINOIC ACID

Up to now, I have focused on what can be done surgically to treat wrinkling *after* it has occurred. But is there something that can be done to prevent wrinkles, or at least slow down their formation? Avoiding excessive sun exposure and always protecting yourself when outdoors with sunscreens of SPF 15 or better, as I pointed out in Chapter 3, are probably the single most important steps you can take to slow the skin's "aging" process. Recently, however, a prescription vitamin A derivative cream, tretinoin cream (RETIN-A cream), has given us some encouragement in the fight against skin aging.

RETIN-A cream, long considered an excellent prescription topical treatment for acne, has shown some promise in freshening the appearance of facial skin and perhaps even slowing down the formation of fine wrinkles. It appears to accelerate shedding and replacement of new skin cells, and it may even stimulate new collagen formation in the dermis.

Applied *very sparingly* twice weekly to all areas of the face, RETIN-A cream may, according to initial medical reports, tone up skin and make it more radiant and youthful-looking. In some cases, these effects were noticeable in a matter of just two to three weeks. However, in most cases the results are seen gradually, over a one-year period, after which the RETIN-A cream must be continued indefinitely in order to maintain the results. This cream should always be applied about twenty to thirty minutes *after* a gentle facewash, never sooner, or excessive drying and flaking of the skin may result. When used as prescribed, my patients have been quite pleased with the results. The role of RETIN-A cream in the treatment of acne will be discussed more fully in Chapter 15.

Fortunately, long-term use of tretinoin cream has not resulted in any significant adverse effects on the skin. Of course, RETIN-A cream is not a panacea for skin aging, nor should it be considered a substitute for good, daily facial skin care. It does, however, give us reason to hope that better and even more useful topical creams and lotions for slowing or reversing the skin aging process are not far off.

14

Face-lifts, Fat Suction,
and Other
Plastic Surgery

The American Heritage Dictionary of the English Language defines the word plastic as "capable of being shaped or formed, pliable." When some people think of *plastic surgeons*, they envision doctors who possess the skill to almost magically transform their faces, like a sculptor molding plastic into something entirely different. Through the years, novels and movies have contributed to this misconception. How many times have you seen a story line in which a character had plastic surgery done to hide his identity and was given a completely new and wonderful face that was totally different from the one he was born with? Sound familiar? But is it true? Unfortunately, at least for now, the answer is NO. Nevertheless, many cosmetic procedures have been developed over the years that can dramatically improve the way you look. And while they may not make you into a completely different person, they often can make you feel so much better about yourself that you become a different person. For some people it is a fresh start.

In the preceding two chapters, I discussed a wide variety of office-based cosmetic surgical procedures such as the excision of unsightly moles, chemical peels, and ZYDERM collagen injections. The procedures described in those chapters are technically all forms of plastic surgery. In fact, some of these procedures

—the excision of unsightly moles, or dermabrasion for acne scarring, for example—frequently are considered plastic surgery. Such surgery is most frequently performed in the doctor's office. The cosmetic procedures I have chosen to include in this chapter are those which, while they are occasionally performed in the doctor's office, are more frequently done in either the outpatient ambulatory operating suite of a hospital, or in a hospital operating room. Many of them, in fact, require overnight stays in the hospital.

In 1984, over 1.5 million Americans had cosmetic surgery to change their looks. This figure is expected to continue to rise every year. All plastic surgery is not performed by plastic surgeons. In times past, plastic surgery of any kind was entirely in the hands of plastic surgeons; today, many different specialties are involved in cosmetic surgery. Many postdoctoral physician residency training programs, in such fields as otolaryngology (ear, nose, and throat), ophthalmology (eye), oral surgery (advanced dental surgery), and dermatology, for example, regularly include training in cosmetic surgical techniques as part of their programs. As a result, your choices of cosmetic specialties has widened. For example, you may consult an otolaryngologist or a plastic surgeon for a rhinoplasty ("nose job"), or you may consult with a plastic, ophthalmologic, or dermatologic surgeon for a blepharoplasty (eyelid surgery). Now you are probably thinking that choosing the right doctor for your needs has become especially confusing, but rest assured: The well-trained and experienced cosmetic surgeon in any of these specialties is capable of giving you an excellent cosmetic result.

The best way to choose a physician for these purposes is to see some of his or her work. Speak with your friends or relatives who have had cosmetic surgery, and ask them if they were satisfied with their doctor's work and care. While often a good form of recommendation, it is, of course, no guarantee, since every person is different and their problems and needs may differ. The next best way of choosing a cosmetic surgeon is by recommendation from a trusted family physician or internist. These doctors often know who is best qualified for the particular kind of surgery you want. A third, but least satisfactory, way of finding a cosmetic surgeon is to contact your local County Medical Society office for a list of board certified physicians who perform the surgery you wish. In general, be skeptical of anyone who guarantees the results of any surgical procedure or seems to unrealistically downplay any of the possible risks. Be wary of any come-ons for "preventive" cosmetic procedures. No aging process can be truly prevented by any kind of surgery. Cosmetic procedures should be performed when they are actually needed.

Recently, there has been a dramatic increase in the number of big-business cosmetic surgery "mills," some with offices all over the country. Many of these places do heavy TV, radio, and magazine advertising. They promise free consultations, early appointments, fast, same-day service, and cut-rate prices. This all sounds great, but be careful! While the come-ons seem attractive, you must remember that you are playing with your face, and you must live with what you have done for the rest of your life. Furthermore, you may not even get such bargain fees at these places. Often, after you have been lured in by the advertising inducements, you may actually pay premium prices for cut-rate work.

Finally, before you set foot in the office of any cosmetic surgeon, you should carefully examine your motives for cosmetic surgery. You can avoid much unnecessary pain and disappointment after surgery if you take stock of your *attitude before* the operation. You are most likely to be disappointed with cosmetic surgery: (1) if you are unsure or indecisive about wanting a particular procedure; (2) if you aren't ready for it; (3) if you tend to be a perfectionist about all things; (4) if you are seeking surgery only to please others; (5) if you expect the surgeon to be a magician. A plain individual can be made more attractive by cosmetic surgery, but will not be turned into a stunning movie star.

Ulterior motives should not be the driving force for having cosmetic surgery. If they are, you are likely to be quite disappointed. For example, if you hope that looking younger will give you more energy or improve your sex life, you are probably setting yourself up for a fall. In general, individuals who have had a long, burning desire to have some change made, those having surgery to please themselves, and those with more modest expectations for the outcome fare the best. When cosmetic surgery is performed for the proper motivations, body and mind can be helped. For the wrong motivations, both can be hurt.

FACE-LIFTS
(RHYTIDECTOMIES)

Facial aging is a fact of life. Sagging and wrinkling result largely from a combination of your own hereditary tendencies for skin aging, the cumulative effects of sun damage over many years, and your own unique patterns of facial muscle use. Redundancy of the skin, the development of jowls, and loss of facial and neck skin elasticity result from gravity acting upon aging skin. Sagging, redundancy, and the deeper kinds of wrinkles and folds related to them are especially amenable to face-lifting. On the other hand, fine wrinkles, such as those found around the mouth, are less amenable. As you learned in Chapter 13, fine wrinkles may be reduced or eliminated by the use of injectable collagen, chemical peels, or dermabrasion, either alone or in combination.

The complete face-lift, or rhytidectomy, is the basic and most popular surgery for skin aging. The results can be quite gratifying; it usually leaves a person looking five to ten years younger. Face-lifts can accomplish three goals: they can lift and smooth the skin of your cheeks and forehead, remove excess skin and puffiness around the eyes, and eliminate the loose, crepey, or flabby skin of the neck. Face-lifts do not change the basic contours of your face, nor can they restore the contours lost through fat loss under your skin. In short, face-lifts remove excess skin and tighten flabby skin. The beneficial results of face-lifts generally last about five or six years, occasionally as long as ten years. The benefits may be prolonged by avoiding overexposure to the sun and keeping your weight constant.

A complete face-lift is a multistep operation that is routinely performed under general anesthesia. The following summarizes the usual steps involved: First the hair is parted all the way around the scalp, about a half-inch in from the forehead. Next, the intended incision (cut) line is mapped out all along the partline (Figure 6a). The remaining hair is tied to keep it out of the way. As you can see, the incision site is selected so that the surgical scar will ultimately be hidden in the hairline and behind the ears.

Excess skin is then removed from the upper eyelids. Following that, redundant skin and puffy fat are removed from the lower eyelids of both eyes. The remaining details of the eyelid surgery are essentially the same as for a simple blepharoplasty, which is covered later in this chapter.

After the eyelid surgery is complete, the surgeon then makes a long incision along the partline. This incision extends in front and around both ears. Afterward, the skin is freed up from the underlying tissue to a distance of about four inches on either side of the incision line. At this point, the surgeon literally lifts up the skin and pulls it like a mask tightly across the face, trims away excess skin, and then sutures the incision closed (Figure 6b). The entire face is bandaged with pads and gauze, and then covered with an elastic bandage or elastic chin strap. Bandages are removed in twenty-four hours, at which point facial puffiness and bruising are usually present, particularly around the eyes.

During the immediate recuperation period you will experi-

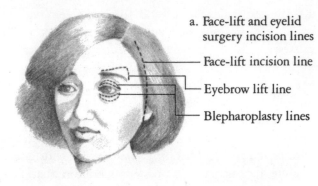

a. Face-lift and eyelid
   surgery incision lines

Face-lift incision line

Eyebrow lift line

Blepharoplasty lines

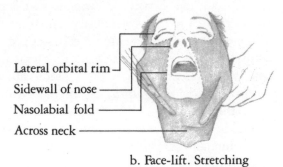

Lateral orbital rim

Sidewall of nose

Nasolabial fold

Across neck

b. Face-lift. Stretching
   skin taut and trimming
   excess away

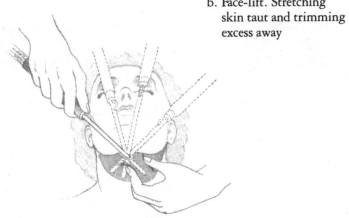

c. Suction lipectomy

FIGURE 6.

ence little pain until the nerves of sensation that were cut during the operation reunite. Afterward, you might feel a "pins and needles" sensation that generally precedes the return of normal sensation. This period of time may last for weeks to months. In general, you will only need to remain "in hiding" for about three weeks after the procedure, but if you tend to be an easy bruiser, you may need to remain in hiding considerably longer. You will be able to wash your hair within three days and will be able to use makeup between two to four weeks after surgery.

Contrary to popular belief, there seems to be no limit to the number of times that face-lifts may be performed on the same person, nor does a masklike face develop after repeated face-lifts. Face-lifts also don't hasten deterioration of facial skin, as some mistakenly believe. Furthermore, having had a face-lift does not prevent you from having other cosmetic procedures, if needed, such as chemical peels or collagen injections.

Clearly, rhytidectomy is a major cosmetic procedure. It usually costs between two and three thousand dollars and requires time off from work. For those reasons, many people opt for many of the other, less radical cosmetic procedures discussed earlier, such as injectable collagen, or more limited forms of cosmetic surgery, such as a blepharoplasty, discussed later in this chapter. On the other hand, with proper attitude, motivation, and preparation before surgery, and with proper support after surgery, the results of face-lifts can be quite dramatic.

Mini-face-lifts

A mini-face-lift is a procedure that has little, in my opinion, to recommend it, except that it is a minor surgical operation, and is therefore less expensive, less uncomfortable, and less inconvenient than a complete face-lift. Mini-face-lifts consist of removing a triangle of skin from above the hairline area of the temples on both sides of the head. The edges of the skin are then pulled and stretched upward and then stitched together. For the upper two-thirds of the face, little cosmetic improvement can be expected from this type of operation. Some improvement is achieved for the lower third of the face, but it is usually short-lived.

Blepharoplasty

Blepharoplasty is an operation designed to correct baggy, droopy, and puffy eyelids. Crow's feet, the wrinkle lines that radiate from the outer corners of the eyelids onto the cheeks, do not respond as well to blepharoplasty. As I mentioned earlier, cosmetic eyelid surgery normally is part of the complete face-lift procedure. However, many patients under forty-five who don't want the discomfort of a full face-lift, or who don't wish to invest the time or the money, can realize significant enhancement in their appearance by simply having blepharoplasties performed. Blepharoplasty generally imparts a brighter, more rested look to the eyes, and thereby can brighten the whole face.

Blepharoplasty consists of making incisions in the folds of both eyelids, removing the redundant skin, and then suturing the remaining skin tightly together (Figure 6a). The incision lines are carefully selected so that after healing is complete, the resulting fine, thread-like scars blend almost imperceptibly with the surrounding skin. In summary, for each lid, excess fat and skin are cut away and the remaining skin is restitched with very delicate suture material to minimize the chance of developing any visible scarring. Blepharoplasty generally takes between one and two hours to perform.

After the operation, the eyelid will be very swollen and black and blue. Despite the appearance, there is usually little postsurgical pain. Swelling and discoloration usually substantially subside within ten days to two weeks. Cover-up makeup may be used at that time. Other cosmetic procedures, such as chemical peels, if needed to enhance the overall esthetic effect, can be performed about three months later. Blepharoplasties usually cost between one thousand and fifteen hundred dollars.

Eyebrow Lifts
(Superciliary Lifts)

Eyebrow lifts can be combined with a blepharoplasty or may be performed separately. Eyebrow lifts are designed to eliminate drooping brows, which can make your eyes look much smaller, or sometimes even prevent you from being able to completely open your eyes. In severe cases, drooping of the outer ends of the eyebrows can cause the upper lids to bulge so much that the lids may even rest upon the eyelashes.

Usually performed under local anesthesia, eyebrow lift surgery simply consists of surgically removing a crescent like piece of skin from the temple area above each eyebrow (Figure 6b) and then suturing the sides of the wounds together. The largest amount of skin is removed at the outer one-third of the crescent, so that when the ends of the wounds are stitched together, the eyebrows are pulled taut and lifted. The stitch lines are oriented so that after healing, the fine, linear scars that result are concealed from view in the eyebrows. Not only do eyes appear larger after brow lift surgery, but crow's feet wrinkles at the outer corners of the eyes may also be slightly improved. Eyebrow lift surgery usually takes about one hour.

RHINOPLASTY
("NOSE JOBS,"
NOSE RESHAPING)

The nose is one of the two so-called "character features" of the face (the chin being the second). *Rhinoplasty* is the medical name for the surgical procedure to correct nasal deformities. In this procedure, excess nasal bone or cartilage is removed, and the nose is then rearranged and reshaped. While rhinoplasty is usually performed for cosmetic reasons, it may be done to alleviate breathing or sinus obstruction problems. Repair of a deviated nasal septum is often combined with rhinoplasty. Long or hooked noses, humped or bumpy noses, wide or thick-tipped noses are among the most common kinds of cosmetic problems that can be benefited by rhinoplasty. Enlarged pores on the nose or thick, oily skin are not improved by rhinoplasty.

"Nose jobs" are usually performed under local anesthesia, although occasionally general anesthesia is used. The incisions and manipulations are performed on the inside of the nose. In many cases, no external cutting is required and there is no external scarring. However, when the nostrils require narrowing, tiny incisions are made on the sides of the nose. Hidden within the skin folds on both sides of the nose, the fine incisional scars usually become imperceptible within a few weeks.

Hospitalization is usually brief. Generally you enter the hospital the night before surgery and leave the day following surgery. Depending upon the complexities of individual circumstances, rhinoplasties require between one and two hours to perform.

After surgery there is usually quite a bit of swelling of the nose, cheeks, and eyelids. Bruising of the eyelids is also common. The nose is frequently packed and splinted after surgery. Packs and splints are removed in a few days. All dressings are usually off by the end of the first week. Most people can return to work in one to two weeks following the surgery. Since, in most cases, no external incisions of the skin are made, makeup may even be used within a few days after surgery. However, eyeglasses may only be worn if special lifts have been placed on the frames to prevent them from resting on the nose, or if they are taped to the forehead. Contact sports should be avoided for three months.

While most of the swelling is gone in four to seven days, it usually takes about twelve months for all the swelling to disappear. Nasal stuffiness may even persist for several months. Right after the dressings are removed the nose will appear somewhat rigid and excessively turned up due to postoperative swelling. As the postoperative swelling disappears, the nose will begin to assume its eventual shape. This usually occurs by about six months. The cost of an uncomplicated rhinoplasty may range from twelve to eighteen hundred dollars.

Rhinophyma

I cannot leave the subject of noses without discussing one special type of disfiguring skin condition of the nose, *rhinophyma*. Rhinophyma is a condition where the oil glands of the nose become markedly overgrown, giving rise to a bulbous, lumpy, bumpy-looking, W.C. Fields-like nose. Rhinophyma usually accompanies severe cases of adult acne (*acne rosacea*, which is discussed in Chapter 15) and occasionally may be the only manifestation of that condition. Rhinophyma can be successfully treated by dermabrasion, and the carbon dioxide laser has also been reported to be successful in treating the problem.

MENTOPLASTY (CHIN AUGMENTATION, CHIN REDUCTION SURGERY)

As I mentioned earlier, the second "character feature" of the face is the chin. Three basic types of defects of the chin are amenable to cosmetic surgical correction: the protruding chin, the elongated chin ("witch's" chin), and the recessive chin. Together, the surgical procedures designed to improve these conditions are referred to as *mentoplasties.*

Chin Augmentation

The most common of all chin abnormalities for which people seek correction is the recessive chin or "weak chin." Occasionally, the presence of a weak chin first becomes noticeable following a rhinoplasty. It seems that in some cases the correction of one defect makes the presence of another more noticeable. In those cases, obtaining the proper facial proportions or balance between character features hinges upon correcting both nasal and chin defects.

For over two decades, the use of silicone implants to augment recessed chins has been the mainstay of cosmetic chin surgery. The silicone in these prostheses is in a biologically inert solid form, and should not be compared with injectable liquid silicone droplets used for wrinkle elimination. While injectable liquid silicone droplets *have* been used in the past for treating moderately or minimally recessed chins, I generally do not recommend this form of treatment for the reasons cited in Chapter 13.

Following the administration of local anesthesia, the surgeon makes an incision either on the inside of the mouth, between the lip and the teeth, or into the skin underneath the chin. Underlying tissue is then pushed aside so that a pocket may be created in front of the natural chin. The silicone prosthesis is then sewn tightly into the pocket. The procedure takes about one and a half hours.

Postoperative discomfort is minimal and recovery is rapid after chin augmentation. In most cases, an overnight stay in the hospital is all that is required. Some people temporarily complain of a slightly artificial feel to the new chin, but this seldom remains a problem.

Chin Reduction

Following local anesthesia, incisions are made either between the lower lip and the teeth inside the mouth, or on the underside of the chin externally. However, instead of inserting a prosthesis, as in chin augmentation, the surgeon chisels off excess bone from the natural chin until its size and proportions are considered esthetically correct. The postoperative course is about the same as for chin augmentation.

OTOPLASTY
("EAR PINNING")

Otoplasty, the operation for correcting ear deformities, is one of the most common forms of aesthetic surgery. Otoplasties are generally used to correct the shape or contour of the external ear. Protruding, "flyaway," or "Dumbo" ears can be the cause of embarrassment and emotional pain. Otoplasty restores the ears to their proper esthetic relationship with the face and head. The results of surgery are quite gratifying.

Otoplasties are usually performed under local anesthesia. Incisions are made behind the ears. Enough underlying cartilage is thinned or removed to be able to position the ears closer to the head. The incisions are then stitched closed. The resulting thin scar is easily concealed within the skin folds behind the ears. Finally, an elastic pressure dressing is placed "turban"-style around the head and ears to hold the ears in place. The operation usually takes between one and three hours, depending upon the individual circumstances and whether the earlobe must also be reduced in size.

The elastic compression dressing is removed in seven to ten days. In general, two or three days of hospitalization are usually required for otoplasties. Most people are able to return to work within one week following the surgery. Swelling and discoloration of the ears and surrounding skin are to be expected and last several days. During the recovery period, eyeglasses need to be modified so that they don't place any pressure upon the ears. For two months following the surgery, a nighttime elastic pressure bandage must be worn.

LIPO-SUCTION
(SUCTION LIPECTOMY,
FAT SUCTION)

Suction has been in use for the removal of localized accumulations of fatty tissue and fatty deformities of the body since its introduction in Europe in the 1970s. It was introduced in the United States in 1982. Since that time, as greater experience has been gained, the technique of *suction lipectomy* has undergone a number of modifications and improvements. In theory, suction lipectomy is like vacuum cleaning. The surgeon uses a thin, blunt, tubelike, "vacuum cleaner-type" instrument called a *suction cannula*, by which unwanted fat is permanently sucked out from under the skin. It is currently believed that once the unwanted fat is removed by lipo-suction, regardless of any future changes in diet or exercise routines, it is gone for good. So far this has proven true in the relatively short time that lipo-suction has been performed. Longer term follow-up is needed, however, to be certain of this.

Lipo-suction has been successfully used to remove unwanted fat from necks, cheeks, "double" chins, and jowls. Lipo-suction of the face is usually an outpatient procedure. Local anesthesia is used to numb the sites of cannula insertion (Figure 6c). To remove fat from the neck area, the cannula is inserted through a small incision made under the chin. The cannula is then swept around in all directions to "vacuum" out the unwanted fatty tissue. For removing fat from the cheeks and jowls, the cannula is inserted through a small incision made below the earlobe. Following suction lipectomy, the small incisions are stitched and the resulting scar ultimately becomes almost unnoticeable. In many cases, the cosmetic results of suction lipectomy have been quite gratifying. More recently, lipo-suction has been combined with face-lift procedures to enhance the cosmetic results. The surgery usually requires thirty to sixty minutes to perform.

Postsurgical discomfort tends to be minimal. Tenderness and bruising are common, and usually last about one week. For several days the skin may feel as though it has been heavily massaged or even "rolled down a hill." An elastic pressure dressing is usually left in place for one week after the procedure. Occasionally, a feeling of numbness in the treated areas follows surgery. It may persist for quite some time, but most often disappears. The cost of suction lipectomy of the face usually ranges from one thousand to two thousand dollars.

Before concluding this chapter, I must reemphasize the point that cosmetic surgeons are not magicians. On the other hand, many different surgical methods are currently available to help you look and feel better about yourself. If you decide to use any of them, make sure your motives are clear and your expectations realistic. Finally, as you go through the operative and recuperative periods, you should bear in mind an aphorism that one very well-known plastic surgery textbook suggests should be appended to the standard preoperative patient instruction sheet for cosmetic surgery: To be beautiful, one must suffer (at least a little and for only a short time).

15

Treating Acne
and Rashes

The purpose of this chapter is not to bore you with a lengthy medical discussion of all the diseases and conditions that can plague your face and scalp. Nor is it my intention to exhaustively review all the different types of medical therapies available to treat them. Instead, I've elected to provide an overview of several of the more common kinds of facial skin eruptions, and to discuss some of the more commonly prescribed medications and treatments for these conditions.

ACNE

In Chapter 7, I discussed in some detail the causes of acne and many of the myths and misconceptions that surround it, and covered some of its better known aggravating factors. In order for you to treat yourself, specific nonprescription medications were recommended and general skin care advice was given. You might wish to refresh your memory by skimming that section again. Unfortunately, not everyone's acne condition improves with self-therapy, despite a diligent regimen of all the recommended steps and the use of all the appropriate nonprescription medications. If you have a persistent, or moderate-to-severe-acne problem, you should consult a dermatologist.

A wide variety of oral and topical prescription medications are available that, when used according to your dermatologist's specific instructions, can help clear up your acne. Your doctor may even combine these medications with some of the nonprescription items that you may have already been using. Unless you are specifically advised differently, the general skin care steps and cosmetic recommendations for caring for acne-prone skin outlined in Chapter 7 should still be followed. And, of course, if you have questions, you should discuss them with your doctor.

Benzoyl Peroxides

Benzoyl peroxides are used to promote peeling, to kill bacteria, and to prevent the formation of the acne follicle plugs. Prescription benzoyl peroxide preparations are invariably gel formulations, whereas most nonprescription benzoyl peroxides are in creams or lotions. Gel forms may be alcohol-based, acetone-based, or water-based, and these are considered more effective preparations than the cream- or lotion-based forms. Those with an alcohol base tend to be the most drying, and those with a water base, the least.

As a rule, products with higher concentrations of benzoyl peroxide usually cause more drying and peeling and are prescribed when more peeling is needed. I seldom prescribe the higher concentration products since additional peeling seldom results in a significant improvement in acne and generally only makes the skin feel drier and more uncomfortable.

Irritation from benzoyl peroxides is not uncommon. Dryness and chapping frequently result from overzealous use of benzoyl peroxides, or the use of an unnecessarily high concentration of benzoyl peroxide, or the use of a product with an overly drying base, such as alcohol. As with any medication, if irritation should occur, discontinue use of the product and consult your doctor.

A large selection of prescription benzoyl peroxide gels

are available. Some of the more commonly prescribed are: BENZAGEL-5 gel, BENZAGEL-10 gel, PANOXYL 5 gel, PANOXYL 10 gel (alcohol-based); PERSAGEL 5 gel, PERSAGEL 10 gel (acetone-based); and PANOXYL AQ2, ½ gel, PANOXYL AQ5 gel, PANOXYL AQ10 gel, DESQUAM-X-5 gel, DESQUAM-X-10 gel, PESA-GEL W5 gel, and PERSA-GEL 10 gel (water-based). Your doctor will choose the particular strength and formulation based upon your special needs. In general, I prefer to start most of my patents on a water-based 2½ percent benzoyl peroxide gel since they are generally the least irritating.

Tretinoin
(Retin-A Cream, Vitamin A Acid)

In Chapter 13, I mentioned the use of tretinoin cream (RETIN-A cream, vitamin A acid) in connection with its recently appreciated ability to retard or reverse some aspects of skin aging. However, the original and still primary use of tretinoin is in the treatment of acne, where tretinoin has certainly demonstrated itself in the judgment of many to be one of the most effective anti-acne topical prescription remedies available.

Follicular plugging is the basis of all acne blemishes. Tretinoin penetrates into the follicles and appears to reverse follicle plugging in two ways: It makes the cells within the plug less sticky, and it speeds the production and turnover of new cells. Benefit from its use usually occurs somewhere after three to six weeks of use. Many people experience a slight worsening of their acne about two weeks after beginning RETIN-A preparations. It is important that you remember this in order to prevent needless discouragement.

RETIN-A preparations come in gel, liquid, or cream forms. All RETIN-A preparations have a tendency to be irritating and to cause some redness or peeling, especially if not properly used. In general, gels are the most drying and creams the least drying. RETIN-A cream should be applied *very* sparingly and no sooner than twenty to thirty minutes after facewashing, in order to minimize its tendency to overdry and irritate the skin. Since sunlight can increase the irritating effects of RETIN-A cream, protect yourself with an SPF-15, nonacnegenic sunblock (Chapter 3) during the warmer months.

Topical Antibiotics

It is felt that the bacterial organism, *Proprionobacterium acnes*, has long played a part in acne development. This is the reason that oral antibiotics, particularly tetracycline (discussed later in this chapter), were the mainstays of acne treatment for over thirty years. Nevertheless, physicians were aware that when they treated acne with oral antibiotics, they were forcing the whole body to be subjected to a systemic antibiotic and its potential side effects.

Fortunately, within the past decade, topical antibiotics specifically formulated for treating acne have been developed. Their effect is limited to your skin, so the potential problems of taking systemic oral antibiotics are largely avoided. Many cases of acne that previously would have required systemic antibiotics (although by no means all) may now be treated with antibiotic lotions, creams, and ointments.

Antibiotic lotions, which are usually alcohol-based, are generally more drying than creams or ointments. If you suffer from acne, but also have dry skin that is easily irritated, your doctor may prescribe a more moisturizing cream- or ointment-based preparation, rather than a drying lotion. On the other hand, if your skin tends to be greasy, the more drying alcohol lotions are usually better. Cream and ointment antibiotics are also ideal for the wintertime when chapping and dryness commonly cause skin to flake and crack. All antibiotic lotions should be applied twenty to thirty minutes after facewashing to minimize the drying effect.

Most dermatologists include topical antibiotics as an important part of their anti-acne regimes. Three chemically different types are most often prescribed: clindamycin, erythromycin, and tetracycline. Most dermatologists feel that topical clindamycin and erythromycin are more effective than topical tetracycline. They may even be as effective as oral tetracycline.

Some of the more popularly prescribed commercial preparations are: CLEOCIN-T lotion (clindamycin); STATICIN lotion (1 percent erythromycin), ERYDERM lotion, T-STAT lotion, and ERYMAX lotion, and AKNE-MYCIN OINTMENT (2 percent erythromycin); TOPICYCLINE lotion (tetracycline), and MECLAN cream (a tetracycline derivative). Most of the lotions come with roll-on applicators for convenience. However, the applicators tend to become clogged and dirty, so if that happens, simply remove the applicator top and apply the lotion with your fingertips. The recently introduced ERYCETTE lotion comes in easy-to-carry erythromycin (2 percent pledgets, each wrapped in a sterile aluminum foil packet).

Oral Antibiotics

Oral antibiotics are believed to affect the same steps in the process of acne formation as topical antibiotics. The three most frequently prescribed oral antibiotics for acne are tetracycline, erythromycin, and minocycline. Since the advent of topical antibiotics and other more effective topical anti-acne medications, oral antibiotics are now usually reserved for treating more severe cases of acne, i.e., those characterized by the presence of highly inflamed pimples, pustules, abscesses, and deep cysts.

Contrary to popular belief, oral antibiotics do not cure acne overnight. As you already know, no medicine currently available can cure acne. Second, oral antibiotics do not work nearly as quickly for controlling acne as they do for curing infections. Ordinarily, you will not begin to see any response to them for about three weeks. Maximal responses to oral antibiotics generally require about six to eight weeks of therapy or longer. Once satisfactory improvement is achieved, oral antibiotics can be continued for maintenance, if necessary, for months or even years.

Fortunately, three oral antibiotics commonly used for acne have few serious side effects. However, minor side effects, common to all of them, can be quite annoying. Vaginal yeast infections (*candida, monilia*) are common, especially when oral antibiotics are taken for prolonged periods; in addition to suppressing the growth of unwanted acne bacteria, the normal bacterial inhabitants of the vagina, which usually keep vaginal yeasts in check, are also suppressed. The vaginal yeasts subsequently overgrow and cause yeast infections. When it is essential for you to be maintained on oral antibiotic therapy, your doctor may prescribe both topical and oral anti-yeast medicines along with the antibiotic, either as a prevention or treatment of yeast infection.

Gastrointestinal upset and queasiness frequently result from taking oral antibiotics, particularly during the first few days of therapy. Often these symptoms disappear if you continue to take the medicine regularly. Diarrhea is another very common complaint, and one that often necessitates stopping the antibiotic for a while and switching to another.

As I mentioned earlier, tetracycline, which comes in capsule form, has been the oral antibiotic of choice for over thirty years. Hundreds of thousands of people with acne have been successfully treated with it through the years. It works, is relatively inexpensive, comes as a generic, and may be taken safely for long periods of time. Tetracycline is effective in relatively low doses and is concentrated in the sebaceous follicles where it is needed. Dermatologists most frequently recommend starting doses of 250 mg four times daily. Once satisfactory improvement is achieved, the dose and frequency of tetracycline are usually decreased or discontinued altogether.

On the down side, tetracycline interacts and becomes less effective when it comes into contact with the calcium, magnesium, or aluminum contained in dairy products and antacids. For this reason, tetracycline must be taken either one hour before or two hours after eating, never along with meals. Since tetracycline usually must be taken four times daily, medication scheduling can become most inconvenient. Many people get fed up and stop taking the drug before it can have any beneficial effects. For the sake of practicality, I usually instruct my patients to take 500 mg of tetracycline twice daily, a routine that is usually just as effective as the four-times-daily regimen, but is far more convenient. However, tetracycline must never be taken during pregnancy since fetal bone abnormalities may result.

Erythromycin is the second drug of choice for acne therapy. It, too, is effective, inexpensive, and may be prescribed as a generic. Erythromycin comes in tablet or capsule forms. Dosages and side effects are much like those of tetracycline. Some people who do not respond to tetracycline, or experience side effects from it, may respond favorably to erythromycin. A variety of commercial erythromycin preparations are available, some of which are supposed to be less irritating to the gastrointestinal tract. Two popular ones are EES-400 tablets, and ERYC capsules, which are supposed to be released in the small intestine (rather than the stomach) where they are less irritating.

Minocycline (MINOCIN capsules and tablets, VECTRIN capsules and tablets) is a tetracycline derivative that appears to be very effective in treating patients who don't respond to either tetracycline or erythromycin. Even though minocycline is a derivative of tetracycline, there appears to be no cross-resistance with tetracycline. The usual dose for acne therapy is 50 mg twice daily, but 100 mg twice daily is occasionally needed for adequate control in more difficult cases. Generally, once control is achieved, minocycline is gradually lowered to a maintenance dose of 50 mg daily or is discontinued entirely. Dizziness, nausea, and vomiting are occasional side effects of minocycline, especially when it is given in higher doses.

Accutane (Isotretinoin, 13-cis Retinoic Acid)

In my opinion, ACCUTANE capsules, an oral vitamin A derivative, represent the single most dramatic recent advance in

systemic anti-acne therapy. It seems primarily to suppress sebaceous gland activity, and this suppression has been shown to
last for up to four months after ACCUTANE capsules have been
discontinued. Furthermore, many people treated with ACCUTANE
capsules have remained free of their acne problem for years
following its use. When I discuss the use of ACCUTANE capsules
with my patients, I usually explain to them that ACCUTANE
capsules for the treatment of severe acne seems to be what
penicillin must have been for the treatment of bacterial infections when it was first introduced—a kind of wonder drug.

Unfortunately, ACCUTANE is *not* for everyone. They have
many potential side effects and are therefore now recommended *only* for those people with severe, scarring, cystic acne
who have not responded to the most aggressive forms of topical
and oral anti-acne therapies. Some physicians occasionally do
prescribe ACCUTANE capsules for individuals with less severe
forms of acne, but I don't agree with this practice, for I feel
that the potential risks outweigh the potential benefits.

The most common side effects of ACCUTANE capsules are
extremely dry skin and severely chapped lips. Occasional nose-
bleeds, soreness of the gums, body aches and pains, itching,
fragile skin, increased sun sensitivity, peeling of the palms and
soles, and increased sensitivity to contact lenses are other common adverse reactions. Most of these side effects clear within a
few days to a few weeks after treatment is stopped. Most important, *you should not take* ACCUTANE *capsules if you are trying to conceive, are already pregnant, or are nursing.* Human
birth defects apparently have been caused by ACCUTANE taken
during pregnancy.

Several more serious, albeit rare, side effects may occur with
ACCUTANE. These are abnormal bone changes in the spine, decreased night vision, changes in mood, blurred vision, hair loss,
and elevated blood lipid (fat) levels. In some cases, these
effects may be permanent, particularly if the drug is not stopped
soon enough.

The dosage depends upon the patient's weight. It is usually

taken twice daily with meals. A full course of ACCUTANE capsules consists of four to six months of daily therapy.

So-called "low-dose" ACCUTANE capsule therapy has been tried in some people and has resulted in satisfactory acne control. However, the beneficial effects of low-dose therapy appear to be comparatively short-lived after treatment is stopped, in contrast with the more lasting effects of the high-dose therapy. I therefore seldom recommend low-dose therapy for my patients.

A small number of people have seen their acne worsen during the first few weeks of ACCUTANE capsule therapy. In general, most people start to see significant improvement after ten to twelve weeks. If necessary, a second course of therapy may be initiated eight weeks after a first course has been completed. Again, for patients with severe, scarring, cystic acne who have not been well-controlled on conventional therapies, ACCUTANE capsules offer a chance for long-lasting relief that simply did not exist before.

Estrogen-Progestin Combinations

The use of birth control pills to control acne goes back more than two decades. As you may recall, the male hormone in both men and women is responsible for stimulating oil gland secretion. In acne therapy, the female hormone estrogen is used not to suppress the ovary, but to suppress male hormone production from the adrenal glands. Likewise, progestational hormones (progestins) interfere with male hormone activity and thus also lead to diminished oil gland secretion.

Years ago, when birth control pills commonly contained higher estrogen contents, many people taking the pill experienced significant improvement in their acne. Owing to concerns about possible estrogen-stimulated breast and uterine cancers, the estrogen content of most currently available oral contraceptives is now considerably lower. As a result, the effect of oral contraceptives in controlling acne is more variable; some people improve with their use while others may worsen.

I generally do not recommend the use of birth control pills for the purpose of treating acne. First, there are many other safe and effective topical anti-acne preparations. Second, I prefer not to tamper with the body's delicate hormonal balance by adding hormones.

It is an entirely different matter if you are already using birth control pills for contraception. In that case, if your doctor feels it is necessary, he or she may switch you to an oral contraceptive that can both serve to protect you against conception as well as help treat your acne. When used for treating acne, it is important to use contraceptive pills with a higher estrogen content, such as ENOVID E, ENOVID 5, and OVULEN.

Acne Surgery

Acne surgery is the technical name for two procedures that your dermatologist may perform: *comedone extraction*, and *incision and drainage of cysts*. I have long maintained that acne surgery is one of the most essential forms of acne therapy. Topical and oral medications generally require several weeks to work, and most people find the wait discouraging. By contrast, the beneficial effects of acne surgery frequently can be appreciated within two to three days, and can provide quite a lift for the acne-weary individual.

Comedone extraction, the treatment of choice for removing whiteheads and blackheads from your skin, not only makes you look better, it prevents the progression of whiteheads to more inflamed pimples, cysts, and abscesses. The procedure is usually performed with a very fine scalpel or with a special instrument called a comedone extractor.

Incision and drainage of cysts is the second form of acne surgery. Here, selected acne cysts and abscesses are opened with a fine blade scalpel and their contents are allowed to drain to the surface. Draining cysts frequently speeds their healing and reduces the risk of scarring.

Most people have two questions about acne surgery: Will it

hurt? Will it leave scars? It *can* be uncomfortable and sometimes even painful, but the results are worth it. If you have a particularly low pain tolerance, your doctor may suggest the use of nitrous oxide (laughing gas) to make you more comfortable during the procedure. As far as leaving scars, when properly performed by a professional, the answer is no. In fact, by preventing whiteheads from progressing to inflamed cysts, your doctor is actually preventing potential scarring.

Therapeutic Injections
(Intralesional Corticosteroids)

The therapy of choice for treating cystic lesions is the injection of an anti-inflammatory agent directly into the acne cysts. The drug most often used for this purpose is triamcinolone acetonide suspension, a corticosteroid. Acne is an inflammation, not an infection as some people mistakenly think. The injection of the anti-inflammatory triamcinolone suspension into acne cysts or abscesses results in their rapid shrinking and resolution. With the low concentrations and the small amounts necessary, the injected suspension basically works just where it is needed; little gets absorbed into the rest of your system.

Most inflamed acne cysts, particularly ones in an early stage, will flatten and disappear within two to three days after injection. It is usually best to contact your doctor as soon as possible after any cysts appear, or even when you just feel them getting started under the surface. The longer an acne cyst smolders in your skin before treatment, the more likely it is to leave a permanent scar. Sometimes a slight depression occurs at the treatment site. This usually disappears in a few weeks, but occasionally requires several months to plump back to normal.

From time to time, patients are reluctant to have therapeutic injections because of the stories surrounding the use of steroids. Steroids, which are used in the treatment of many conditions, unquestionably have side effects. These side effects, however, usually occur when a person receives large daily doses of steroids orally or by injection for many weeks or months, for chronic conditions such as rheumatoid arthritis or systemic lupus erythematosus. Since little of the steroid in the therapeutic injections for acne is actually absorbed into your body, there is little basis for concern.

Acne Rosacea (Rosacea, "Adult Acne")

No discussion of acne for adults would be complete without covering the subject of adult acne or *acne rosacea* (or *rosacea*). To the thirty-, forty-, or over-fifty-year-old woman who asks me when she is finally going to outgrow her "teenage" acne, I often respond that she is no longer suffering from so-called "teenage acne," but from "adult acne."

Rosacea is a chronic problem that affects the central oval of the face and neck, and that can be both medically and cosmetically quite troubling. Acne pimples, pustules, and cysts are a prominent part of rosacea. Whiteheads and blackheads are characteristically absent in rosacea. In fact, the absence of whiteheads and blackheads is a helpful sign to your dermatologist that he or she is dealing with rosacea and not common acne.

Rosacea is a complex condition, however, that not uncommonly consists of more than just acne. People with rosacea may be prone to prolonged episodes of facial flushing, to the formation of numerous "broken" blood vessels, and to the development of overgrown oil glands (*sebaceous hyperplasia*) on the face and nose. In extreme cases (more frequently in men), overgrowth of oil glands on the nose may lead to a W.C. Fields-type nose (rhinophyma, see Chapter 14). In addition, eyelid margin irritations (*blepharitis*) and other eye problems may accompany rosacea.

Diet can play a significant role in some cases of rosacea, unlike in acne vulgaris. Alcohol, caffeine-containing beverages, such as coffee, tea, and colas, hot temperature beverages, extremes of heat and cold, and spicy foods have all been felt to aggravate rosacea. If you notice a relationship between any foods and your condition, you should either eliminate that food from your diet or cut its intake down drastically. For example, if you are a ten-cups-of-coffee-a-day person, reduce the coffee to your best two cups of the day. Finally, increased nervous tension and excessive sun exposure also aggravate rosacea, as they do common acne.

The treatment of rosacea depends upon the individual circumstances. The acne component of rosacea can be treated just like common acne, although for rosacea the single most important and effective therapy seems to be the use of antibiotics, particularly tetracycline or minocycline. If "broken" blood vessels or overgrown oil glands become cosmetically distressing, they may be treated with electrosurgery (see Chapters 12 and 13). If rhinophyma occurs, it may be treated with dermabrasion (Chapter 13). Eye problems, if present, may require consultation with an ophthalmologist.

Perioral Dermatitis

Perioral (around the mouth) *dermatitis* is a relatively common acne-like condition that affects primarily women in their twenties and thirties. The eruption consists of many small pimples and pustules arranged in clusters located around the mouth, on the sides of the nose, and on the chin—the so-called "muzzle" area. The skin directly around the lips is usually spared.

While the cause of perioral dermatitis is not known, many cases are presumed to result from the use of topical corticosteroids on the face. Other possible causes are the use of fluorinated toothpastes, certain fragranced cosmetics, and the birth control pill.

Therapy for perioral dermatitis is gratifying. The patient must discontinue contact with any possibly inciting substances and take oral tetracycline or minocycline. With initiation of appropriate therapy, the perioral dermatitis usually clears completely in one to two months. A second course of tetracycline is occasionally necessary.

COMMON FACIAL RASHES

Seborrheic Dermatitis
(Seborrheic Eczema)

Seborrheic dermatitis, a form of eczema that involves the face and scalp (as well as other body areas), is a very common, recurrent skin rash. Seborrheic dermatitis usually affects those areas of the face having the highest concentrations of sebaceous glands, namely the eyebrows, between the eyes, around the nose, and in and around the ears. On the face, seborrheic dermatitis usually appears as pinkish-yellow rounded spots or patches, with thin, greasy scales on top.

Seborrheic dermatitis can take several forms. Simple dandruff of the scalp, the most common cause of embarrassing flaking and itching, is one familiar form. When seborrheic dermatitis is more severe, large areas of redness and flaking may develop, as well as patches of scaly, thick crusts throughout the scalp. These spots and patches can be quite itchy and cosmetically distressing.

The cause of seborrheic dermatitis is not known. A hereditary tendency to develop it seems to exist. Increased nervous tension or physical stresses certainly can aggravate the predisposition. If you are overweight, diabetic, or have a neurologic condition called *Parkinson's disease*, you may also be more troubled by seborrheic dermatitis. Diet is of little importance. Seborrheic dermatitis is a condition that has spontaneous ups and downs. It is not contagious.

Although there is no known cure for seborrheic dermatitis, your dermatologist can do much to control its symptoms and improve your appearance. For milder cases of the scalp, your doctor may simply recommend the use of commercial antidandruff preparations. Zinc pyrithione, sulfur, salicylic acid, and tars are the most commonly recommended active ingredients in antidandruff shampoos.

For more severe cases, 2 percent selenium sulfide shampoos, such as EXSEL medicated shampoo and SELSUN medicated shampoo, seem to work best. Where shampooing alone does not control your problem, your doctor will probably prescribe one of a number of topical corticosteroid lotions or gels. Of the many available preparations, I suggest TOPICORT GEL, LIDEX GEL, and DIPROSONE lotion. They penetrate well into the scalp where the problem originates, and they generally do not make hair greasy or difficult to style.

If you have a mild or moderate seborrheic dermatitis of the face, prescriptions containing hydrocortisone 1 percent or 2.5 percent, in vanishing cream bases, usually clear up the condition in a few days. SYNOCORT cream and HYTONE cream are two of the most popularly prescribed brands of hydrocortisone creams. For more severe cases of the face, higher potency topical steroid preparations may be temporarily needed to bring the condition under control.

Once satisfactory control is achieved, your doctor may recommend one of a number of different lotions, creams, or ointments containing sulfur, salicylic acid, sodium sulfacetamide, or tars for maintenance therapy. Unlike the case with topical corticosteroids, these other medications can be used for long periods of time with no adverse effects upon your skin. On the other hand, prolonged use of high potency topical corticosteroids may result in premature, irreversible thinning and wrinkling of the skin. A topical corticosteroid cream may look and feel like an ordinary cold cream, but it should never be used like one. Topical corticosteroids are *potent topical medications* with potential adverse side effects. They should be used with caution, only when needed, and under a doctor's supervision.

Rather than relying on available commercial products, I prefer to individualize a person's maintenance medication by having the pharmacist compound a preparation to order for each of my patients with seborrheic dermatitis. This way I have more control over the particular ingredients in the preparation, their concentrations, and the type of bases into which the active ingredients are dissolved. In other words, I can more easily vary the kinds and amounts of the active ingredients to suit a particular patient's changing needs and circumstances.

Psoriasis

Psoriasis is a chronic disorder that affects between three and five million Americans, and nearly 3 percent of the world's population. Psoriasis may involve any or all areas of the body, including the nails. For the purposes of this book, however, I am only concerned with psoriasis of the face and scalp. In psoriasis, skin cells are produced about seven times more rapidly than normal. Instead of being shed easily, like normal skin cells, they stick together to form thick, crusty spots. Psoriasis is not contagious.

Heredity appears to play a significant role in who develops psoriasis. Clearly, it runs in certain families. The first attack may occur anytime from birth onward, and a number of aggravating factors are known to trigger or worsen psoriasis in the genetically predisposed individual. Injuries to the skin, such as cuts, scrapes, surgical wounds, excessive skin dryness and irritation, sore throats, increased nervous tension, and certain medications such as lithium or propanalol, have all been known to set it off.

In its most typical form, psoriasis of the face and scalp appears as reddish spots or patches covered by thick, adherent, whitish scales. If the scales are removed for any reason, pinpoint bleeding areas will be seen underneath. Psoriasis can occasionally cause itching, and can be a source of severe cosmetic embarrassment.

Unfortunately, no cure for psoriasis is currently available, although satisfactory treatment is possible. Your dermatologist may treat you with many of the same preparations discussed earlier for treating seborrheic dermatitis. In addition, since most cases of psoriasis improve following ultraviolet light exposure, your physician may recommend that you gradually expose yourself to sunlight, when seasonally feasible, or suggest the use of artificial ultraviolet light sources, when sun exposure is not possible. However, I prefer to prescribe other methods to control psoriasis, since, as I emphasized in Chapter 3, ultraviolet light exposure can result in premature aging of the skin and the formation of skin cancers.

If your patches of psoriasis are thick and scaly, you might be given a salicylic acid preparation such as KERALYT GEL or SALIGEL to thin them out. Thinner patches permit deeper penetration of topically applied creams and lotions. Intralesional injections (injections given directly into the psoriasis patches) of triamcinolone, like those used to treat acne, are also useful in treating psoriasis. Intralesional injections are particularly effective for people with particularly resistant patches of psoriasis or those with only a few patches.

Finally, anthralin, a petroleum derivative long used to treat psoriasis, has enjoyed a recent upswing in popularity. At one time anthralin formulations were greasy and messy, and were notorious for staining both clothing and skin. For those reasons, it fell into disfavor with most patients. Recently anthralin has been reformulated in a vanishing cream base. For the scalp, the anthralin product I prefer is DRITHO-SCALP cream, and for the skin, either DRITHO-CREME or LASAN'S CREAM.

Regardless of which psoriasis treatment your doctor prescribes, once you achieve satisfactory control or clearing, make it a daily routine to use a thick moisturizing cream or lotion on your face in order to prevent dryness and irritation (which could prompt another psoriasis flare-up).

Atopic Dermatitis (Atopic Eczema)

Atopic dermatitis is another very common condition, affecting about 3 percent of the U.S. population. Most outgrow it but for certain people the problem is lifelong. Atopic dermatitis occurs in individuals with either a family or personal history of asthma, childhood eczema, hay fever, and hives.

Excessive use of soap and water, rapid swings in temperature, excessive exercising with profuse sweating, woolen clothing, periods of heightened emotional and physical stress, such as overwork, fatigue, colds, sore throats, and allergy attacks may bring on atopic dermatitis. Occasionally certain foods, such as citrus fruits, may aggravate it in some people.

Atopic dermatitis can assume a variety of forms. It usually manifests itself in dry, brownish-gray, scaly, and thickened patches on the cheeks, darkish rings about the eyes, and accentuated lines under the eyes. In more acute forms, lesions of atopic dermatitis may redden, blister, weep, and crust. Further, atopic dermatitis can involve any area of the body; seldom is the condition limited to the face. The itching that accompanies it can be quite distressing, even incapacitatingly disruptive, particularly at night.

Exceptionally dry skin almost always goes hand in hand with atopic dermatitis. Not uncommonly, people who suffer from it are particularly sensitive to many different types of cosmetics.

Mild to moderate atopic dermatitis of the face, like seborrheic dermatitis, responds well to mild corticosteroid creams. For cases where symptoms are severe or there is pronounced facial and eyelid swelling, a short course of oral corticosteroids, such as prednisone or dexamethasone (DECADRON), may be needed.

Antihistamines, used alone or in various combinations for their anti-itch and sedative benefits, often are needed also. ATARAX, DURRAX, SINEQUAN, ATAPIN, and BENADRYL are among the most commonly prescribed brands of antihistamines. Unfortunately, a common side effect of most of them is drowsiness. However, after several days of continuous use, a number of people become acclimatized to the antihistamines and continue to enjoy relief from itching, but no longer feel drowsy.

Once your atopic dermatitis is satisfactorily under control, make every effort to keep your skin well-lubricated. Dryness is one of your worst enemies, and it must be avoided, for it often paves the way to recurrences. If you are aware of any particular foods that aggravate your condition, by all means avoid them. However, be aware that skin tests for food allergens, and desensitization shots, like those used for hay fever, are of limited value in atopic dermatitis. I therefore don't routinely recommend them to my patients.

Contact Dermatitis (Contact Eczema)

Contact dermatitis is yet another form of eczema. However, unlike those already mentioned, contact eczemas are not linked to heredity, nor are they aggravated by physical or emotional stress. They are simply allergies or irritations that develop in response to a substance applied to the skin. If contact dermatitis comes on suddenly (*acute* contact dermatitis), you will see redness, swelling, blisters, weeping, and crusting. If it has been going on for a while (*chronic contact dermatitis*), your skin will become thickened, cracked, and blotchy in color. Contact dermatitis is typically very itchy.

If your rash is determined by your dermatologist to be strictly the result of a physical irritation—rather than a true allergy—the rash is termed *irritant* contact dermatitis. Solvents, caustic chemicals, and industrial strength soaps and detergents are notorious for causing this type of rash. The rashes of irritant and allergic contact dermatitis can often appear quite similar. However, unlike allergens, physical irritants are able to provoke rashes on the first exposure, while allergens generally require at least one prior exposure to your skin before provoking the rash.

Most cosmetics and topical medications manufactured today are tested to be sure that they seldom cause direct irritation when applied to the skin. If an allergy should result, however, it is referred to as *allergic contact dermatitis.* No matter, how "hypoallergenic" a particular cosmetic is supposed to be, there are usually some people who will become allergically sensitive to it.

Table 2 lists five groups of common causes of contact dermatitis of the face and ears. If you are wondering why hand creams and nail care cosmetics are included, the answer is that almost anything that gets on your hands invariably is transferred onto your face and eyelids. For years, in fact, the most common cause of contact dermatitis on eyelids was nail polish.

In the case of true allergic contact dermatitis, your first brush with the culprit allergen almost never results in a rash; it may be the second, third, tenth, or even hundredth exposure that will finally bring it on. Therefore, what may *seem* to you like the sudden onset of an allergy may have actually taken days, weeks, or sometimes even years to develop.

Treatment for contact dermatitis is simpler than for the other forms of eczema. If you are able to isolate the culprit allergen and make every effort to avoid further contact with it, the rash will gradually disappear. In more severe cases, however, you may need medical treatment to alleviate your symptoms and reduce the swelling. The therapy is generally the same as for atopic dermatitis.

To prevent future attacks of allergic contact dermatitis, it is extremely important, of course, to avoid the use of any products you suspect are troublemakers. To determine which product you are allergic to, follow the steps described in Chapter 4.

Unfortunately, many products developed for the same purpose have a number of the same chemical ingredients in their formulations. For example, *parabens* (preservatives) are found in many different brands of creams and lotions. Therefore, unless you specifically find out the exact ingredient in a particular product that causes your allergy, you may have to avoid all products of that kind. When you have no idea which specific product of the many you may be using is causing your problem, your dermatologist can perform special allergy tests, or patch tests, to isolate the specific allergen.

TABLE 2

COMMON CAUSES OF
CONTACT DERMATITIS

1. *Hair sprays, shampoos, hairdyes*

2. *Jewelry, ear appliances,
and foreign objects*

3. *Cosmetics, soaps, perfumes,
hand creams, nail care cosmetics*

4. *Topical medicaments*

5. *Plant resins
(poison ivy, oak, sumac)*

Patch tests consist of challenging your skin with a screening series of the most common potentially allergenic ingredients contained in most cosmetics, medications, jewelry, etc. Test materials are placed on Band-Aid-like patches and taped in place on your back or inner arms, where they are left undisturbed for a minimum of forty-eight hours. Unlike scratch testing, with which it is often confused, patch testing requires no breaking of the skin and is entirely painless.

A patch test is considered positive if redness, irritation, or itching develops at any site within forty-eight hours, and a positive test means that the specific culprit has been identified. Your doctor will then be able to give you the ingredient's common and trade names. Armed with this information, you can examine every product label to be sure that you don't accidentally purchase any products that contain that ingredient.

On the other hand, if you already know which product you are allergic to, your dermatologist can help you find the specific ingredient that is causing it. In many cases, the doctor is able to obtain from the manufacturer test samples of each of the ingredients contained in the product and can administer the patch test to discover the specific troublemaker allergen(s).

16

Treating Hair Loss

Alopecia is the medical term for hair loss. In Chapter 9 you learned some common causes of temporary and permanent alopecia and some ways for recognizing and dealing with them on your own. However, there are times when medical intervention is necessary. In this chapter I discuss the steps the dermatologist follows in order to diagnose hair loss problems, and the medical and surgical treatments available for dealing with hereditary hair loss (*androgenetic alopecia*).

Diagnosing a particular alopecia problem can sometimes prove quite difficult. To thoroughly investigate the possible cause of any hair loss condition, your doctor must weigh all the information obtained from your complete medical history, a physical examination of the hair and scalp, and the results of blood and hair tests.

To obtain a complete medical history, your doctor will ask you a wide variety of questions pertaining not only to the hair loss condition, but also to your recent general health. Your doctor will want to know whether your parents or other close blood relatives have a significant hair loss. You will be questioned about the ways you routinely care for your hair and scalp, and what medications, if any, you take for other medical conditions. The answers to these questions are extremely helpful in pinpointing the causes of a hair loss problem. For example, in families where hair loss is common, a hereditary basis for alopecia would have to be strongly considered.

Knowing exactly how you routinely treat your hair and scalp is likewise extremely important. You will recall, for example, that having your hair "permed" too frequently, especially if it is dyed, or overusing tight rollers, to name just two types of potentially damaging hair care practices, can result in hair fragility and breakage, situations that can resemble true alopecia.

Certain physical and emotional stresses on the body, such as childbirth, high fevers, surgery, and crash diets can be causes of temporary hair loss. The answers to questions about the regularity of your periods and changes in hair distribution on your body, such as whether you have recently noticed increased facial hair growth or have to shave more frequently under your arms, may suggest to your doctor the presence of a glandular (*endocrinologic*) problem.

In addition, many medications can be responsible for hair loss. These include birth control pills, COUMADIN and heparin (blood-thinning drugs), INDOCIN (anti-inflammatory drug), TEGRETOL and TRIDIONE (anticonvulsants), INDERAL (heart and blood pressure medication), lithium carbonate (agent for controlling manic-depressive illness), allopurinol (gout medicine), and a number of anticancer drugs. In most cases, early discontinuation of the culprit drug usually results in complete regrowth of hair.

In "working up" hair loss, the dermatologist will carefully examine your hair and scalp, paying special attention to such things as the texture of your hair, its length, and the pattern and distribution of the hair loss. He or she will also search for any evidence of infection, inflammation, scarring, or tumorous growths, all of which may contribute to alopecia.

Depending upon the leads suggested by your medical history and physical examination, your doctor may order certain blood or hair tests. Most frequently, specific blood tests are ordered to determine whether you are suffering from anemia or iron deficiency (*complete blood count, Serum Iron and Total Iron Binding Capacity*), thyroid abnormalities (*T3, T4, and TSH levels*), or overproduction of male hormones (*plasma testosterone levels*). Certain forms of anemia and iron deficiency, overactive (*hyperthyroidism*) or underactive (*hypothyroidism*) thyroid conditions, and other glandular (*endocrine*) problems of the adrenal glands and ovaries have all been associated with hair loss. Additional tests may also be required under certain circumstances. For example, if infection is suspected, specific cultures will be obtained and an ultraviolet light examination (*Wood's Light*) for fungus infection may be performed.

A variety of hair tests are frequently needed to evaluate hair loss problems. These are the Hair Pull Test, Hair Clipping Test, Hair Pluck Analysis, Three Week Hair Collection, Hair Shave Examination, and Scalp Biopsy. It is unlikely that your doctor will perform all these tests, since there is considerable overlap in the kinds of information derived from them. I have found the Hair Pluck Test, Three Week Hair Collection, and occasionally the Scalp Biopsy to be the most consistently useful.

The *Hair Pull Test* is performed by simply running the fingers through the hair. Abnormal hair loss is considered present if ten or more loose hairs are collected in this way. The shafts of the collected hairs are then examined to determine whether the majority of them are growing hairs or resting hairs.

The *Hair Clipping Test*, as its name implies, is performed by clipping between ten and twenty hairs at the surface of the scalp. The procedure is painless. The hairs are then examined under the microscope for any abnormalities of the hair shafts and hair cuticles.

The *Hair Pluck Test* is a quick, albeit momentarily painful, pluck of between twenty and fifty hairs from the scalp. A rubber-tipped clamp is used to grasp the hairs, and a temporary burning sensation immediately follows. The plucked hairs are examined under the microscope to determine the specific types of hairs present, the ratio of growing to resting hairs, and the existence of any structural abnormalities of the hair shafts.

The *Three-Week Hair Collection* involves gathering up hairs you lose in the sink, shower, or bath drains, and on your pillow or clothing. I always tell my patient that this test is a *feasible* hair collection because no one can be expected to collect all the hairs they shed during the three weeks, even if they are extremely diligent about it. Each week's collection is packaged in an envelope and labelled appropriately.

Many patients with hair loss understandably come to the dermatologist fearful that they are losing hair so rapidly that they will soon be bald. But they tend to overestimate the number of hairs they lose each day. Most of them are not even aware that a person with no hair loss problem normally loses between 50 and a hundred hairs each day. Hence the Three-Week Hair Collection is one of the best ways a doctor has to assess just how many hairs are actually lost each day. I have also found that forcing people to make the hair collection is one of the best ways to reassure them that they are actually not losing the number they thought they were. When a person is experiencing a heavy hair fall, repeated Three-Week Hair Collections may be performed every six to eight weeks in order to determine when the hair shedding has slowed or ceased.

The *Hair Shave Examination* technique can be useful for determining both hair density (the number of hairs per square inch of your scalp) and the rate of hair growth, and it helps the dermatologist evaluate the frequent complaint, "My hair doesn't grow." For this test an area of one square inch is shaved on the right side of the head. First the density of the hairs is measured, and measurements of growth rate are periodically made as hair grows back. Hair ordinarily grows at a rate of about one-quarter to one-half inches per month. Women who dye their hair need not have any area shaved, because the rate of hair growth can be determined by measuring the growth rate of the untinted hair.

Finally, a *Scalp Biopsy* may be required to confirm a suspected diagnosis or when additional information is needed to establish a possible diagnosis. (Scalp or skin biopsies are discussed in greater detail in Chapter 17.)

A Scalp Biopsy is simply a minor surgical procedure in which the doctor removes a small piece of scalp tissue and sends it to a pathologist (microscopist) to be analyzed for evidence of inflammation, scarring, the presence of tumors, and sometimes for infections. In some cases, the pathologist may even be able to determine whether *androgenetic alopecia* (common hereditary hair loss) is the cause of the problem.

Chemical hair analysis involves a battery of chemical tests on a collection of your hairs to analyze them for their content of specific proteins and chemicals such as selenium and sulfur, and heavy metals, such as lead, mercury, and arsenic. However, in the evaluation of hair loss, chemical hair analysis is generally felt to be of little value. The tests can also be quite expensive.

The finding of deficiencies or excesses of certain chemicals in the hair doesn't necessarily mean that you need to modify your diet. In fact, the results of chemical hair analyses frequently do not correlate well with actual body content or nutritional requirements of these chemicals. Chemical hair analysis has found its best use in detecting the presence of a heavy metal poisoning, such as lead, but its routine use has no place in the investigation of common hair loss problems or nutritional problems.

ANDROGENETIC ALOPECIA
(MALE/FEMALE
PATTERN BALDNESS)

Many people mistakenly believe that only men are at risk of balding, and still others believe that the tendency for balding is inherited only from the father. To set the record straight, both men and women can bald, and the tendency for balding may be inherited from the parent of either sex. Moreover, since androgenetic alopecia is genetic in nature, and since doctors are unable at present to alter your genes, no cure for androgenetic alopecia yet exists. Nevertheless, treatments for hair loss are available and new methods are constantly being developed to deal with this problem.

It is believed that androgenetic alopecia or common male/ female pattern baldness is caused by a heightened sensitivity in genetically susceptible individuals to male hormones called *androgens*, which are produced by both men and women. The patterns of male and female balding, however, do differ. A receding hairline at the temples or a central area of baldness on the crown of the head, the so-called "monk's cowl," are typical of male pattern baldness. Male balding, which can begin as early as age twenty, may progress until all but a small fringe of hair on the back and sides of the head remains.

Female pattern alopecia follows a different progression. Genetically predisposed women notice a gradual and diffuse thinning of the hair over the entire scalp sometime between puberty and their forties. In general, female alopecia is more pronounced toward the top front of the scalp. While very few women progress to total baldness as men do, they may still lose sufficient numbers of hairs to diffusely expose large areas of scalp, and this can be quite troubling.

Hair Transplantation

Developed more than a quarter of a century ago, hair transplantation is primarily used to surgically treat select cases of male pattern baldness. Less commonly, hair transplantation is also used to treat several other types of hair loss problems. Basically, the process entails transferring (*transplanting*) healthy hair follicles from an area of more dense hair growth to a region of less dense growth.

Hair transplantation is only occasionally used to treat select cases of female pattern alopecia. This is because hair transplantation is generally better suited to treating the nonuniform pattern of male baldness than to the diffuse pattern of female hair loss. The reason: You cannot really expect to see any net improvement in appearance if you transfer hair from one area of diffuse hair thinning to another. This contrasts sharply to the situation in men where transferring hair-bearing plugs of scalp from a region of relatively dense hair growth to a completely bald area results in a substantial cosmetic improvement because of the net gain in hairs in the bald area. Nevertheless, hair transplantation surgery may be helpful for treating selected cases of androgenetic female alopecia, especially where the hair loss has been patchier than usual.

Some people respond negatively to the first suggestion of hair transplantation surgery. For some, the word *transplantation* has a frightening connotation; others confuse it with the surgical hair replacement technique called *hair implantation*, which has gotten much deserved bad press. (A medically frowned upon procedure, its dangers are discussed later in this chapter.)

Hair transplantation surgery is basically quite simple. After clipping and pinning the hair, the *donor* area (the area from which the plugs containing healthy hair follicles will be removed) and the *receptor* area (the bald area into which the plugs will be transplanted) are anesthetized with local anesthesia. A circular "cookie-cutter"-like instrument called a *punch* is used to cut out plugs of bald scalp in the receptor area. This can be performed manually or with an electric drill. The bald plugs are discarded, leaving circular openings in the scalp. The same punch is then used to bore out plugs from the donor area. Each donor plug may contain between six and twenty healthy hair follicles, depending upon the original density of the hair in that area. These plugs are then inserted into the receptor holes and oriented to give a natural appearance to the hair growth. Anywhere from forty to approximately a hundred plugs may be transplanted in one session.

The wounds are cleaned and, if necessary, some of the donor sites are stitched together to control bleeding. However, most donor site wounds are usually left to heal by themselves. Small scars will ultimately form at the donor sites and no hair will ever again grow there, but these site scars will be well-concealed by the surrounding hair. After the procedure, the scalp is wrapped in a turban-like pressure bandage dressing, which is usually worn for about twenty-four hours.

After the procedure, there may be some pain and swelling, but these problems usually last no more than twenty-four to forty-eight hours. A scab soon forms a crust over each transplanted plug. These crusts generally fall off about two to three weeks later.

The hairs that were present within the transplanted plugs at the time of the surgery do not themselves grow. Instead they fall out within a few weeks after the procedure, as a response to the stress of surgery (a form of telogen effluvium. See Chapter 10). However, four to five months after the transplantation surgery, new, healthy hairs begin to grow in the transplanted plugs.

Additional hair transplantation surgery may be performed at four- to eight-week intervals. The use of different-size donor plugs for filling in sites contributes to a more natural look. The total number of hair transplantation procedures that may be performed is limited by the density of the hair at the donor sites. Enough hair must be left within these areas to adequately cover the donor site scars. In other words, thickening of the recipient areas cannot be done at the complete expense of the donor areas.

Hair transplantation gets its name from the fact that hair follicles are being *grafted* (*transplanted*, moved) from a hair-bearing area to a bald area. Hair transplantation neither stimulates nor grows new hairs. Therefore, after hair transplantation, you will *not* have more hair than you had before. You are simply making better use of the hair that you do have, i.e., the doctor is only moving your hairs to an area where they will do more cosmetic good.

The average cost of hair transplantation surgery currently ranges from fifteen to twenty dollars per plug. In the properly selected patient, the cosmetic results can be quite satisfactory. Unfortunately, not everyone is a good candidate for hair transplantation. If you are considering it, discuss the pros and cons in detail with your dermatologist. If you do decide to have it done, avoid cut-rate hair transplantation "clinics" for the same reasons mentioned in the last chapter for plastic surgery "mills." From some of these so-called clinics, you'll be lucky to escape with your hair.

Scalp Reduction and Flaps

In some women, though it is rare, there is a bald spot so large and sparse that the donor area would have insufficient numbers of plugs to adequately cover it. In this instance, the surgeon may choose to perform *scalp reduction surgery* prior to hair transplantation. (A very large bald area, however, usually cannot be removed without damaging the blood supply to the area.) Using local anesthsia, a major portion of the bald patch is simply cut out to reduce its overall size. Following scalp reduction, the smaller bald area may be transplanted in the usual manner. The obvious advantage of scalp reduction surgery is that many fewer donor plugs are needed to fill in the surgically reduced recipient area.

Like hair transplantation, rotation of a *pedicle flap* is another method of putting your own healthy hair, from a normal, denser part of your scalp, to better advantage. In this procedure, instead of using donor plugs, a large, thick flap of hair-bearing scalp is partially cut free from the scalp, and left attached to it by a "stalk" (*pedicle*). The bald recipient area is completely removed. The hair-bearing flap is rotated around on its stalk to cover the bald area and then stitched into place. Like hair transplantation, no new hairs are being created. The hair you do have is merely repositioned into a location where it will serve the most cosmetic good.

Hair Implantation

Hair implantation basically consists of *sewing* human hair into the scalp. Anchoring stitches or wires are first placed into the scalp, after which a hairpiece or tufts of hair are firmly attached to the anchoring stitches. The dramatic appeal of this technique is its guarantee of a full head of hair in an instant. That part is certainly true. On the other hand, the risks and complications of hair implantation far outweigh any benefits.

With today's technology, most commonly used suture materials, although "foreign" to the body, cause little irritation when left in place for the short periods of time required for the healing of most surgical wounds. However, in the case of hair implantation surgery, where the anchoring stitches are intended to remain within the scalp indefinitely, the body frequently becomes intolerant of their presence; the scalp may become inflamed, extremely tender, or a painful infection with pus formation and drainage may follow. In time, the infection can work loose the anchoring stitches, and they are extruded from the scalp. Severe scarring can result, and even irreversible destruction of the surrounding, previously healthy hair-bearing regions can occur. Victims may require months of intensive systemic antibiotic therapy to cure the infections. Since it is extremely difficult to locate and remove all of the anchoring stitches, their continued presence in the scalp prolongs these problems.

Even in those cases where there has been little or no scalp reaction, the benefits of hair implantation appear to be short-lived. Routine daily hair grooming eventually loosens and finally pulls out the anchoring stitches. The anchoring stitches ordinarily are loosened in about one year, though occasionally it may take as long as three years. Finally, it is also difficult to properly care for your scalp and natural hair under the stitched-on hairpiece, and scalp problems can result.

My advice is to stay away from hair implantation.

Minoxidil

Minoxidil, a potent drug for dilating blood vessels, has been used for some time to treat high blood pressure that is resistant to other medications. Many patients taking minoxidil noticed growth of unwanted hair on various parts of their bodies. These observations led to a tremendous amount of research into the topical use of minoxidil to treat baldness. When minoxidil is in lotion form and applied topically to the scalp only a little, if any, is believed to be absorbed into the general system. Used in this way no unwanted hair growth occurs elsewhere on the body. However, until further studies are conducted, the FDA is *cautioning* against its routine use in alopecia treatment.* Exactly how minoxidil works in treating alopecia is not known, but it may dilate the blood vessels in the hair follicles and prolong the mature growing phase of the hair follicle.

While exciting and promising, the results of using topical minoxidil have not been as dramatic as one might wish. Nonetheless, evidence to date, which reflects more than three years of clinical experience in the treatment of alopecia, indicates that topically applied minoxidil stimulates hair growth in a third of balding patients and may even retard hair loss in others. Unfortunately, not all individuals who do experience hair growth have sufficient regrowth of normal mature hairs to make any significant cosmetic difference. In some cases, the hair that grows is too short and fine (immature hairs).

The best candidates for a trial of topical minoxidil therapy are young people who have only recently experienced hair loss and have relatively small thinning areas. Individuals who have a fair amount of residual, fine immature hairs (*vellus hairs*) in the sparse areas are also more likely to enjoy success. In general, minoxidil works better for restoring hair on the top of the head than near the hairline.

Even in ideal candidates, hair growth does not usually begin until about three to four months after therapy—it is applied to

---

*Six individuals recently were reported to have died while concurrently applying minoxidil for hair loss. No conclusive evidence exists, however, directly linking minoxidil to these deaths, although caution is being advised until more is learned.

the scalp twice a day—has been started, and sometimes it may take as long as six months. If you and your doctor agree that a trial of minoxidil might be worthwhile in your particular case, plan on expending the time, effort, and money for *at least four months.* Then, if new hair growth is ultimately stimulated, topical minoxidil applications must be indefinitely continued at least once daily in order to sustain the new growth.

The use of topical minoxidil is currently an expensive proposition, though a commercial preparation is scheduled to be marketed in the near future. It is supposed to be more reasonably priced. At present, however, pharmacists must compound minoxidil lotions by dissolving the powder obtained from minoxidil capsules into various types of solutions. For this service, most pharmacies have been charging between eighty and two hundred dollars for a four- to six-week supply, depending upon the potency of the lotion. Considering that you must wait at least four months before you even know whether minoxidil will work for you, it can be a pricey gamble.

All in all, minoxidil is by no means a panacea in the treatment of baldness, but it is unquestionably an exciting first step in that direction. Currently being investigated are other topical drugs that may be even more beneficial than minoxidil. Time will tell.

Hormone Therapies of the Scalp

Since androgenetic alopecia has been related to a heightened, heredity-determined sensitivity to the presence of the male hormones, it is understandable that for years researchers focused much of their attention on hormonal remedies to counteract balding. Topical testosterone, progesterone, and estrogen-containing creams and lotions, as well as injections of estrogen and progesterone, have all been used to reverse hair loss. Each of these hormone treatments had its own therapeutic rationales.

At the present time, despite ardent claims to the contrary, the consensus of medical opinion maintains that hormone therapies can at best occasionally stimulate slight hair growth, but not enough to be of any cosmetic significance. On the other hand, it is very difficult to accurately judge the claims made by some patients or their physicians that hormonal treatments are successful for preventing further hair loss. The rate of any person's hair loss may be so variable from season to season and year to year that it is hard to claim with certainty that any apparent decrease in the rate of hair loss in a particular individual is actually due to the hormone being used, or to that individual's predetermined genetic timetable for hair loss. In other words, it is harder to judge how well a drug (in this case a hormone) can prevent or slow further hair loss, than it is to judge whether it can stimulate hair growth.

The above controversy notwithstanding, the use of hormonal preparations to treat hair loss is not without its risks. Topically-applied testosterone, if absorbed sufficiently through the skin, may have masculinizing side effects in women. Estrogens and progesterones likewise may be absorbed through the skin and can possibly play a subtle role in upsetting the body's delicate hormonal balance. Locally injected progesterone occasionally can be extremely irritating to the skin and is capable of provoking an intense inflammation at the injection site. Furthermore, hormone treatments generally must be continued for long periods of time and so can run into a considerable expense.

When considering any claims for the hair-growing benefits of hormonal creams, ointments, and injections, remember: Hormone therapies have been around for years. If they were truly capable of producing such remarkable results, why haven't they received the same hype as minoxidil? I think the answer is obvious: There really hasn't been much to hype. Until such time as there is adequate medical evidence to support their routine use, I strongly advise against using estrogens and progesterones in any form for the treatment of hair loss.

ALOPECIA AREATA

Alopecia areata is a common hair loss condition that may affect men and women of any age, particularly young adults. A family history of alopecia areata has been found in 10 to 20 percent of those affected. And it frequently occurs in families with histories of asthma, hay fever, eczema, or autoimmune diseases, such as pernicious anemia, Hashimoto's thyroiditis, vitiligo, Addison's disease, and juvenile diabetes mellitus.

Alopecia areata is believed to be an autoimmune disease, one wherein your body begins to attack itself just as it would attack foreign invaders, such as bacteria or viruses. These diseases are a kind of "allergy to self." For reasons that are unknown, in an individual with alopecia areata, the body's immune system acts as though the normal hair follicles were an "enemy" and begins to attack them. This quickly slows down hair production and induces a kind of hibernation of the hair follicles. The hair follicles are not dead; they retain the potential to regrow under certain circumstances, yet in approximately one-third of all sufferers regrowth never occurs.

In alopecia areata, roundish, hairless patches suddenly appear on the scalp. There are usually no other accompanying symptoms. Alopecia areata can range from mild to severe. When the hair loss is extensive, alopecia areata can be the cause of substantial suffering.

Any hair-bearing area of the body may be involved, but the scalp is the most common location. When alopecia areata involves the entire scalp and results in a complete loss of hair, it is referred to as *alopecia totalis*. When hair is lost over the entire body, it is referred to as *alopecia universalis*.

The course of alopecia areata has its ups and downs. In general, the younger the patient at the time the condition begins, and the more widespread the hair loss, the poorer the chances for regrowth. Complete, spontaneous recovery occurs in approximately one-third of all patients, and partial recovery in about another third. Spontaneous recovery may take place within months or years. Repeat attacks of alopecia areata are not uncommon.

Treating Alopecia Areata

The mildest cases of alopecia areata are sometimes treated by the application of a high potency, anti-inflammatory topical corticosteroid cream or ointment. Topical corticosteroids are especially useful in children where repeated injections of cortisone or its derivatives would be too emotionally or physically traumatizing.

For most adults with mild to moderate disease, the most common therapy consists of periodic injections of the cortisone derivative triamcinolone suspension. Multiple little injections are given directly into the skin of the bald patches with an ultrafine needle. Usually these are only mildly uncomfortable, and the individual may even return to work afterward. The injections can be repeated every three to four weeks. Several treatment sessions frequently are required to achieve the desired hair regrowth.

When therapy successfully stimulates hair growth, new hairs first appear within four to twelve weeks as a very fine, downy growth. If no regrowth is seen after three to four treatment sessions, it is usually not worth continuing the injections. Sometimes, the new hairs grow back white. Therapeutic injections to one group of alopecia patches do not prevent the occurrence of new patches elsewhere. Should any new patches appear, they are treated in the same fashion.

Minoxidil

Topical minoxidil has been found more successful in treating alopecia areata than androgenetic alopecia. Between one-third and one-half of the patients with alopecia areata treated in trial investigations demonstrated cosmetically acceptable regrowth of hair with topical minoxidil. It has even been successful in some cases of more extensive alopecia totalis and universalis. Because it is so easy for people to use, it has become my second line of treatment following therapeutic triamcinolone injections.

Irritants and Allergens

Hair regrowth in alopecia areata can sometimes be stimulated by irritating the scalp, with either physically irritating or allergy-provoking substances. Somehow, the irritation is believed to stimulate hibernating hair follicles to produce new hair. ANTHRALIN cream or ointment is one of the most frequently used physical irritants. It is applied once daily to the bald patches and is washed off anywhere from ten minutes to several hours later, depending upon the specific circumstances. When anthralin therapy is successful, new hair growth can be seen about two months after beginning therapy. On the down side, in addition to being very irritating to the skin and causing itching, anthralin temporarily stains the skin a brownish-red color. Therefore, care must be taken to limit its application only to the affected areas to prevent irritation and staining to the surrounding skin.

Dinitrochlorobenzene, poison ivy resin, and *squaric acid dibutyl ester* are three of the substances commonly used to induce an allergic rash in patients with alopecia areata. As with anthralin, it seems that the irritation and inflammation created by these substances in some way rouses the hibernating hair follicles to produce new hair. About half of the patients treated in this way will respond. Even when regrowth has occurred, treatment must be continued indefinitely or until a spontaneous recovery takes place. In general, allergic rashes can be quite itchy and uncomfortable, particularly during the humid summer months, accounting at least in part for the general lack of popularity of this form of treatment.

PUVA

PUVA, which stands for *p*soralen plus long-wave *u*ltraviolet light *A* therapy, is occasionally suggested for treating more severe forms of alopecia areata that have not responded to other therapies. Unfortunately, few patients with alopecia areata respond to PUVA therapy. A light-sensitizing medication, psoralen, is ingested by the patient two hours before exposure to the ultraviolet light. Treatments are given in the dermatologist's office and may be required from two to five times weekly. PUVA therapy is therefore expensive and time-consuming. Given the repetitive exposure to ultraviolet light, even when it works, PUVA's potential long-term risks of inducing premature skin aging and skin cancers must be carefully weighed against its potential short-term benefits.

Oral Steroids

When hair loss in alopecia areata is extensive and progresses rapidly, the dermatologist may recommend the administration of oral steroids, usually *prednisone* or *dexamethasone*. Prednisone and dexamethasone are both synthetic cortisone derivatives. When taken with meals, and used in low doses for short periods (three to four weeks only), oral steroids usually have few side effects. However, since extensive alopecia areata often requires prolonged therapy, the potential side effects of systemic steroids, specifically water retention, weight gain, increased skin fragility, stomach upset and irritation, and bone thinning and weakening become more likely. Moreover, even when hair regrowth is stimulated by systemic steroids, the hair may again fall out once they are stopped. For these reasons, I reserve the use of oral steroids for a very small number of patients with severe alopecia areata (or alopecia totalis and universalis) for whom the more conservative therapies already discussed were found unsuccessful.

National Alopecia
Areata Foundation

Although not actually a treatment for alopecia areata, I could not close this section without special reference to an organization dedicated to helping people who suffer from all forms of alopecia areata. Through its activities, support groups, workshops, and its periodical publication, *National Alopecia Areata Newsletter*, individuals with alopecia areata draw mutual support, find out the latest information on research and hair prostheses, and basically learn to cope. For the address of your local chapter and additional information, write to the National Alopecia Areata Foundation, P.O. Box 5027, Mill Valley, California 94941.

There are a number of other less common inflammatory and scarring hair loss conditions such as *lichen planopilaris, chronic discoid lupus erythematosus*, and *pseudopelade of Broca*. A discussion of these conditions is beyond the scope or intent of this book. Many of the diagnostic tests and procedures discussed in this chapter, as well as many of the treatments described for androgenetic alopecia and alopecia areata, however, are also used to diagnose and treat these rare conditions.

17

Curing Precancers and Skin Cancers

In Chapter 3, you learned about the skin's public enemy number 1—the sun—and that the sun can cause not only premature aging and wrinkling, but precancerous and cancerous skin growths, especially if there is a hereditary tendency.

Skin cancers pose both a medical and a cosmetic problem for your skin. They can become quite disfiguring. Between five and fifteen thousand people annually die from skin cancer, and thousands more are disfigured by the partial or total loss of eyes, ears, noses, and lips. This chapter focuses on the various kinds of common malignant skin *neoplasms* (growths), how the doctor diagnoses them, and what he or she can do to rid you of them.

In the United States, approximately half a million people develop skin cancer each year, and one out of every seven Americans is estimated to develop some form of skin cancer during his or her lifetime. These statistics make skin cancer the most prevalent form of cancer; and the incidence of skin cancers, particularly melanoma, appears to be rapidly rising. Fortunately, the majority of them can be prevented by simple avoidance of excessive sun exposure and liberal, topical use of sunscreen and sunblocking agents when sun exposure is unavoidable.

In general, skin cancers are named after the cells of the epidermis that give rise to them. *Carcinoma* is the medical word for cancer. If you refer back to Figure 1, you will recall that the epidermis is composed of several different cell types: squamous cells (middle and thickest layer of epidermal cells), basal cells (most of the bottommost row of cells), and melanocytes (interspersed between basal cells in the bottommost row). If squamous cells become malignant, the resulting tumor is called a *squamous cell carcinoma.* If basal cells become cancerous, the neoplasm is called a *basal cell carcinoma,* and if melanocytes become malignant, the resulting cancerous growth is called a *melanoma.*

Each type of cancer begins when a single cell becomes abnormal. In most cases, the damaging ultraviolet rays of the sun are primarily responsible for initiating this change. Once the change has occurred, the abnormal cell begins to grow and divide in a rapid, uncontrolled fashion. Figure 7 illustrates how precancers and cancers begin. Skin malignancies can appear anywhere on the body, but not surprisingly they occur most commonly (90 percent of the time) on sun-exposed areas, i.e., the face, neck, arms, and back.

To make life a little more confusing, dermatologists have more than one name for the same kind of skin malignancy. For example, squamous cell carcinomas are sometimes referred to as *epidermoid carcinomas* or *intraepidermal carcinomas.* Basal cell

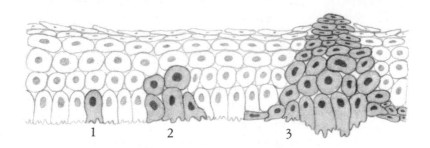

FIGURE 7. Development of skin precancers and cancers from a single abnormal cell

cancers are sometimes called *basal cell epitheliomas*. In each case the terms are synonymous and doctors often use them interchangeably.

Nearly all the premalignant and malignant lesions discussed in this chapter in some way have been related to overexposure to the sun. For basal cell and squamous cell skin cancers this relationship is clear and straightforward: Their occurrence is related to the *cumulative* effects of sunlight over many years.

For pigment cell skin cancers, such as melanoma, the relationship to sun exposure is somewhat less clear. Nevertheless, it seems that sunlight is in some way involved. The risk of developing melanoma appears linked to episodes of having been sunburned, particularly during childhood and adolescence. The greater the number of episodes of sunburn, the greater the risk of developing melanoma.

While just about anyone is at risk for developing skin cancer, certain individuals are at higher relative risk. You are more likely to develop skin cancer if you are fair-skinned, fair-eyed, and sunburn easily (i.e., have Type I or Type II skin. See Chapter 3). In general, blondes and redheads, and blue, gray, or green-eyed persons are more susceptible to sun damage because they have less of the sun-protective pigment, melanin.

People with outdoor occupations, or who are outdoor enthusiasts, generally also run an increased risk of developing skin cancers. Farmers, sailors, construction workers, and golfers, among others, are particularly prone. If you live in the sunbelt regions of the South and West, where the sun's rays are normally more intense, you are also at greater risk. Finally, those who have a strong family history for skin cancer formation are more likely to develop them.

Besides sunlight, several other factors have been linked to basal and squamous cell skin cancers. People who have been treated by X-rays, for any reason, such as those having received facial X-rays for acne, are at higher risk. Those who have been exposed to arsenicals, either occupationally or in the form of medications, have also been found to be more prone to skin cancers. Years ago, a popular arsenic-containing elixir called FOWLER'S SOLUTION was used to treat a variety of ailments, especially asthma.

Squamous cell skin cancers are known to arise within regions subjected to repetitive trauma or within chronically scarred areas. Squamous cells which arise within scars or result from prior X-ray treatment tend to be more serious than those that arise in sun-damaged areas. And squamous cell carcinomas that arise within areas of trauma, scarring, previous radiotherapy treatment sites, and on the mucous membranes, such as the lips, are potentially far more serious. They are more likely to spread to other areas of the body through the blood or lymph system (*metastasize*).

While you will probably find it difficult to distinguish a malignant skin growth from the many different kinds of benign skin growths, there are two important warning signals: (1) the appearance of any new growth, and (2) changes in an old growth, mole, or "beauty mark."

Changes in a growth that may be significant are changes in size, shape, or color; irregularity in outline, loss of surface markings, spreading of pigment outside the confines of the original growth; crusting, bleeding, itching, and pain. Having a growth that fits these criteria does not mean that you definitely have skin cancer; it *does* mean that you should seek professional evaluation by a dermatologist immediately. "Playing ostrich," or following the oft-quoted but mistaken, "if you don't bother a growth it won't bother you" can result in unnecessary delay in obtaining proper medical care. The longer the delay, the greater the potential of serious physical scarring or, even more tragically in the case of melanoma, loss of life.

The American Cancer Society and the American Academy of Dermatology urge you to perform periodic self-examinations of your skin. In a brightly illuminated room, with the aid of full-length mirrors to examine your whole body, use hand-held mirrors to examine hard-to-see places, and a hand-held blow dryer to push away hair in order to see the scalp easily. Examine *all* of your skin and look for the warning signs described above. Particularly in the case of malignant melanoma, early detection offers the best chance for cure.

DIAGNOSIS OF
SKIN MALIGNANCY

Many benign (nonmalignant), harmless skin growths have such characteristic appearances that an experienced dermatologist, simply by examining them with nothing more than a magnifying glass, will have no trouble telling you that they are positively benign and nothing to worry about. However, even to the trained eye, certain growths are difficult to definitely diagnose by visual examination alone. In that case, a biopsy is needed to help establish the precise diagnosis. A biopsy is the only sure way your doctor has of telling you whether or not you have skin cancer.

For some people, the mere mention of the word biopsy often conjures up frightening associations, so I generally avoid using the word with my patients until the biopsy procedure is explained in detail. The word biopsy upsets some people simply because it means that the doctor is entertaining a diagnosis of cancer. Others fear that a biopsy may cause or spread a cancer. *Biopsies do not cause cancer; they merely help the doctor diagnose it.*

Quite simply, a skin biopsy is a minor surgical procedure in which a small piece of skin is removed from a suspected growth and examined under the microscope by a pathologist. A pathologist is a physician specifically trained to recognize abnormal tissues under the microscope. A dermatopathologist is a physician specifically trained to microscopically diagnose skin diseases.

Two main types of skin biopsies are commonly performed —the incisional biopsy, and the excisional biopsy. Which type of biopsy your doctor performs will depend upon the type of growth suspected, its shape and presumed depth. The instruments used for biopsies, and the actual steps involved, are similar to the procedures already described for cosmetically removing various benign growths (See Chapter 12).

An incisional biopsy consists of removing a small piece of tissue (not the whole growth), under local anesthesia, and then sending it to the pathology laboratory for processing and analysis. Your doctor may choose one of five methods to do an incisional biopsy. A *shave biopsy* is an incisional biopsy in which the tissue is "sliced" off with a scalpel. A *curet biopsy* is an incisional biopsy where a superficial scraping is taken from the surface of the suspected lesion. A *scissor biopsy* is a form of incisional biopsy that is ideal for growths in which a large bulk of the lesion projects above the surface of the skin. Taking a *punch biopsy* involves using a "cookie-cutter"-type instrument to remove a deeper piece out of the growth. Punch biopsy is performed when a growth is too large to remove simply for diagnostic reasons and when it is necessary to analyze the deeper portions of a growth. A scalpel, like a punch, can also be used when deeper tissue examination is required. Punch and scalpel biopsies generally require stitches. The other forms do not.

In an excisional biopsy, the entire growth is removed under local anesthesia. Once again, the specimen is sent to the laboratory for processing and analysis. Excisional biopsies are performed when an analysis of the deeper portions of a growth are essential not only for diagnostic considerations, but, in some cases, for estimating future prognosis. Excisional biopsies are frequently performed when a serious skin cancer, such as melannoma, is being considered.

TREATMENT OF
SKIN MALIGNANCY

Skin malignancies may be treated in a variety of ways depending upon the type, its location, the age of the patient, cosmetic considerations, and other factors. Your dermatologist will discuss with you the best treatment alternatives for dealing with your specific problem. Here again, just as with the biopsy procedures mentioned earlier, the details of the surgical cures for skin cancers are similar to the methods described in detail in Chapter 12 for the cosmetic removal of many types of benign growths. Radiation therapy (radiotherapy) and Moh's Chemosurgery, two forms of cancer treatments that have no place in the treatment of cosmetic conditions, are described in the following sections. The most frequently used procedures for curing skin cancers include curettage and electrodessication, surgical excision, and cryotherapy. Under certain circumstances chemical applications may be used.

Radiation therapy (radiotherapy, X-ray therapy) and *Moh's Chemosurgery* are two major forms of skin cancer therapy. At one time used for treating a variety of benign and malignant skin conditions, radiation therapy today is primarily reserved for treating skin malignancies. It is not used for any form of cosmetic work. Radiotherapy, using less deeply penetrating, superficial X-rays, has been successfully used for many years to treat basal and squamous cell skin cancers. Both these forms of skin carcinomas are highly sensitive to the damaging effects of X-rays. Unfortunately, malignant melanomas are relatively radioresistant (radiation resistant), which means that radiotherapy is unsuccessful in treating them.

Shielding all normal skin from the radiation beam, radiotherapy is administered in divided doses (*fractionation*) to the cancerous growth. Treatments are usually spaced over a period of several days. A typical basal or squamous cell carcinoma may require between five and ten individual treatment sessions depending upon the individual circumstances. Treatments may last from seconds to minutes. The patient feels no discomfort and requires no presedation or anesthesia. Basically you feel nothing, as when you have a routine chest X-ray.

After a few treatment sessions the radiation produces destruction of the growth. An intense inflammation develops within the malignancy (the desired effect), frequently resulting in redness, swelling, and pain in the treated area. Complete healing requires a few weeks. The cosmetic results are quite satisfactory and the cure rate is on a par with curettage and elecrodessication—about 97 percent.

Radiation therapy is usually used for people who refuse surgery, for very elderly people for whom surgery would be difficult, and in some cases to treat recurrent skin malignancies. Although the cosmetic results of radiotherapy are initially very good, I generally do not recommend it to young patients; after ten or twenty years radiation-treated areas may begin to show the "weathering" effects of prior X-ray therapy, namely thinning and fragility of the skin, texture changes, and the development of many "broken" blood vessels (telangiectasias). I also don't recommend X-ray therapy for treating skin malignancies on severely sun-damaged areas of the skin. The long-term cosmetic results of treating such areas with radiotherapy can be less than satisfactory. Although in the past most dermatologic radio-therapy was performed by dermatologists in their offices, today most patients are referred to radiotherapists for X-ray treatments.

Moh's Chemosurgery is a highly specialized form of cancer surgery that is particularly effective for treating difficult or recurrent skin cancers. Very large malignancies, and the 3 percent of basal and squamous cell skin carcinomas that recur after other forms of treatment, are best treated by Moh's Chemosurgery.

In brief, Moh's Chemosurgery first involves making a detailed map of the tumor in all its quadrants. This map is used to illustrate the exact location of each section of tissue removed from the malignancy during the procedure. The cancer is systematically sliced out in steps in its three dimensions. After each cut, the Moh's Chemosurgeon repeatedly examines the excised tissue under the microscope to ensure that all the tumor is being removed. For large tumors, Moh's Chemosurgery may require several hours.

When all of the abnormal tissue has been excised, the

wound is left to heal on its own. Stitches usually are not required. Although healing may be somewhat slow, the ultimate cosmetic result is usually quite satisfactory. When a very large area is excised, a skin graft from another location of the body may be required in order to close over the large defect (hole) left by the surgery. The cure rate of Moh's Chemosurgery for treating recurrent basal cell and squamous cell skin cancers is an impressive 96 percent.

PRECANCEROUS GROWTHS
OF THE SKIN

Squamous cell skin cancers and melanomas pass through clinically recognizable precancerous stages. Basal cell skin cancers have no specific premalignant stage that is easily recognizable. In the case of squamous cell skin cancers arising at sites of prior sun damage, precancers are referred to as *actinic keratoses* or *solar keratoses*. The words *actinic* and *solar* both refer to sunlight. The word *keratosis* (plural: keratoses) refers to any condition where there is an excessive growth and accumulation of scaly, horny material. Melanomas have three types of premalignant lesions: the large *congenital nevus*, the *dysplastic nevus*, and *Hutchinson's melanotic freckle*. The following sections describe the various types of precancers and cancers of the skin, as well as their available treatments.

Actinic (Solar) Keratoses

Actinic keratoses appear as red or reddish-brown, often scaly, irregularly surfaced, well-demarcated roughenings of the skin. Occasionally, they may be smooth and flat. Frequently, when numerous, actinic keratoses can stand out quite prominently, particularly on the skin of fair individuals. The diagnosis of actinic keratosis usually can be made by clinical examination alone. Sometimes, however, a shave or curet biopsy may be necessary to clinch the diagnosis. In addition to the visible actinic keratoses on the skin surface, many people frequently have actinic keratoses that are just in the process of forming below the surface. These *precursors* (precancers) are too small to be seen by the naked eye. As a rule, it takes many years for sun-damaged skin to manifest into visible actinic keratoses.

Treatment: Actinic keratoses may be treated variously. Owing to the very superficial location of the actinic keratosis within the skin, a biopsy itself usually removes enough abnormal tissue to be curative. Further therapy is unnecessary.

One form of therapy for actinic keratoses deserves special mention—the topical application of the chemical 5-FLUORO-URACIL (5-FU), (EFUDEX, FLUOROPLEX). It works by specifically interfering with the metabolism of the precancer cells, and 5-FU is primarily used to treat individuals with multiple or numerous actinic keratoses. This form of therapy has the distinct advantage of not only eliminating actinic keratoses that you can see, but of seeking out and destroying those that are just beginning to form below the surface, and are thus not yet visible. Treatment with topical 5-FU can leave your skin much less mottled, much smoother and younger-looking.

However, a course of 5-FU therapy can be a distressing experience for most people, and this is the reason that few people opt to try it after all the details have been explained. Made in cream or lotion formulations, 5-FU must be applied twice daily to the face, though one must be particularly careful to avoid getting any in the eyes, nose, or mouth. In most cases, 5-FU must be applied for between two and four weeks in order for it to be effective. Little happens within the first week of treatment. Sometime between the second and fourth weeks, the actinic keratoses (those visible and those previously invisible to the naked eye) will become extremely red, and finally blister into open sores. There is usually intense burning and pain during this time, for which painkillers and anti-inflammatory corticosteroid creams may be prescribed. Complete healing usually occurs between the fourth and eighth weeks. Occasionally, the combined use of topical 5-FU and corticosteroids is used to try to prevent the brisk inflammation. This therapy has been satisfactory for some people. Nevertheless, for most patients the inflammation, discomfort, rawness of the skin, and the need to be "in hiding" for a few weeks discourage them from opting for topical 5-FU. Despite its immense usefulness, I seldom have occasion to prescribe it in my practice.

Multiple or numerous solar keratoses can be alternatively treated with a full-face trichloroacetic acid chemical peel, such as the kind described in Chapter 13 for the elimination of wrinkles and skin blotchiness. Dermabrasion can likewise be successfully used to treat multiple actinic keratoses. In many cases, both chemical peels and dermabrasions can also eliminate many invisible actinics. As with the topical 5-FU therapy, you must be prepared to hide your face until satisfactory healing takes place.

I find simple curettage under local anesthesia ideal for treating one or a few isolated patches of actinic keratoses. Electrosurgery following curettage is sometimes needed to treat thicker lesions. In general, many of my patients find curettage with or without electrosurgery more convenient and emotionally more palatable than topical 5-FU, or even chemical peels and dermabrasion. With simple curettage, the invisible actinics cannot be treated and must be treated when they appear. Despite that, it has been my experience that most people prefer to return periodically to have their actinics curetted, rather than endure several weeks of topical 5-FU treatment.

Liquid nitrogen (cryosurgery) is another effective alternative method for treating actinic keratoses. Each lesion is touched from ten to thirty seconds with a cotton-tipped applicator soaked in liquid nitrogen. The procedure is fast, simple, and generally satisfactory.

Congenital Nevi (Birthmarks)

The word *congenital* means present at the time of birth. *Nevus* means a mole, or as some people like to call it, a "beauty mark." Therefore, a *congenital nevus* (plural: nevi) is simply a mole that you were born with and not one that developed anytime afterward. About 1 percent of all newborns have congenital nevi. Congenital nevi are grouped according to their sizes: small —less than two-thirds of an inch; medium—between two-thirds and nine inches; and large—greater than nine inches.

The size of a congenital birthmark is very important. The lifetime risk of developing a malignant melanoma in a person with a large congenital mole is approximately 6 percent, compared to only 0.7 percent for a person without a congenital mole. Although precise figures are not yet available, the lifetime risk of developing a malignant melanoma in small and medium congenital moles also seems to be increased as compared to the population at large. Contrary to popular belief, the presence of hair in a mole does not necessarily make it more dangerous.

Treatment: For large and medium congenital nevi, the treatment of choice is complete surgical excision whenever possible and as soon as possible. In this way the pathologist (microscopist) can make certain that the entire growth was removed. For very large congenital moles, where complete surgical excision is not practical, some dermatologists have tried dermabrasion or cryosurgery, but these two methods are not generally recommended, since they cannot guarantee that all congenital mole cells have been completely removed.

Some dermatologists choose to periodically follow their patients with the use of diagrams, photographs, and measurements at intervals of six to twelve months. At these periodic visits, the doctor checks to see whether any of the warning signs of malignant change have occurred. If they have, the doctor will biopsy the suspicious mole. If no changes have occurred, the individual will be seen again in several months.

In general, I recommend prophylactic surgical excision for even small congenital moles. Since melanoma is a very serious and potentially life-threatening skin cancer, I feel that leaving them alone poses unnecessary risks. For a small mole, the excision would be small and the cosmetic result in most cases excellent. Surgical excision eliminates the risk of developing a melanoma in that spot.

Dysplastic Nevi

Much attention is currently being paid to a particular type of mole, the *dysplastic nevus*. The word *dysplastic* means faulty development. Dysplastic nevi may develop anytime after birth, but particularly during adulthood. These moles differ from ordinary moles in several ways. You are all no doubt familiar with the Pap test used by gynecologists to detect *dysplasia* of the uterine cervix, a precursor of cervical cancer. By analogy, a dysplastic nevus is felt to be a precursor of malignant melanoma. It is also felt to be a marker for an individual who has an increased lifetime risk of developing malignant melanoma. That is, people who have dysplastic nevi are not only at risk of developing melanoma within their dysplastic nevi at some point in their lifetimes, but are also at risk of developing melanoma elsewhere on currently normal-appearing areas of their skin.

Dysplastic nevi are usually more numerous than ordinary moles. Young adults generally have an average of about twenty-five ordinary moles on their bodies, and new moles rarely appear after the age of forty. Individuals with dysplastic nevi may have more than a hundred moles and new ones continue to form throughout one's life. Moreover, ordinary moles usually are found on sun-exposed areas and only infrequently on sun-protected areas such as the scalp. Dysplastic nevi occur in many of the same locations as common moles, but, in addition, are often found in unusual locations, such as the scalp. It is estimated that individuals having dysplastic nevi may have a lifetime risk of developing malignant melanoma of between 5 percent and 20 percent, compared to 0.7 percent for the general population.

Dysplastic moles are usually larger than ordinary moles and often have irregular borders. They may range in size from approximately one-quarter to one-half inch in diameter. Dysplastic nevi are usually *flat* or pebbly surfaced, and are frequently variegated in color, displaying shades of tans, browns, and pinks which may fade imperceptibly into the surrounding skin color.

The tendency to form dysplastic nevi seems to run in certain families, although isolated nonfamilial cases do occur. The lifetime risk of developing malignant melanoma approaches 100 percent for people with dysplastic nevi who also have at least two first-degree blood relatives (parents, aunts, uncles, siblings, and first cousins) who have had malignant melanoma, and at least two relatives who have dysplastic nevi. It is of course possible that all cases of dysplastic nevi are familial and that the dysplastic nevi have not yet developed in other family members, but will appear in the future. For these reasons, all close family members of people with known dysplastic nevi should seek dermatologic consultation to have all their moles examined. It could be life-saving. Even if no dysplastic nevi are found at the time of examination, it would be advisable to return at least once every eighteen months for a full skin physical.

Treatment: Any mole that in any way looks atypical should be biopsied. To continue the analogy started earlier between dysplastic nevi and dysplasia of the uterine cervix, a skin biopsy would be analogous to the Pap test to find out if anything is already wrong or going wrong. If a dysplastic nevus is found, I subscribe to the recommendation that it should be entirely excised so that it will never have the opportunity to turn into melanoma. When few dysplastic nevi are present this is feasible. When there are many of them, I recommended that only the most suspicious-looking lesions be biopsied and removed. The rest may be followed by periodic examination of the skin, supplemented by the use of measurements, diagrams, and photographs where appropriate. For those people *without* a family history of melanoma or dysplastic nevi, I recommend follow-up examinations at six-month intervals. For those *with* family histories of dysplastic nevi or melanoma, I advise three- to six-month follow-up visits because of the potentially greater risk of melanoma development in those cases.

Hutchinson's Melanotic Freckle
(Lentigo Maligna)

The last major type of precursor to malignant melanoma is the so-called Lentigo maligna or Hutchinson's melanotic freckle, named after the person who described it. Lentigo maligna is a darkly pigmented, flat spot that mostly occurs on the faces of older people. It is estimated that perhaps as many as one-third of all Hutchinson's freckles progress to malignant melanoma. Hutchinson's freckles usually begin as tannish, freckle-like (hence the name Hutchinson's melanotic freckle) discolorations of the skin that grow larger and change color with the passage of time. They may vary in color from tan to black.

Treatment: Once again, surgical excision is the treatment of choice. Where this is not feasible, X-ray therapy has also been successfully used.

By now you have no doubt realized that the most important message in this entire discussion of premalignant lesions is that having a growth present on your face for many years is no assurance that there is nothing wrong with it. If you have such a growth and it has never given you any cause for concern, it may just mean that you were lucky up to that point. Don't press your luck! See a dermatologist so that if you have some form of precancerous growth it can be removed early, before a real problem begins. It's good preventive medicine, and it's one of the best ways I know to save your face.

SKIN CANCERS

Basal Cell Carcinoma

Basal cell skin cancer is the most common form of skin cancer in white people. It occurs much less frequently in dark-skinned people. Between three hundred thousand and four hundred thousand *new* cases of basal cell carcinoma occur each year. These cancers mostly arise within heavily sun-exposed areas of the skin, such as the head and neck.

As a rule, basal cell carcinomas do not metastasize (spread through your blood or lymph system to other organs of the body), nor does one die from them. Nonetheless, a basal cell carcinoma should not be dismissed as "a little nothing," or a "pimple." It is still a malignant growth and will continue to grow in an uncontrolled fashion. If neglected, it can burrow deeply into your skin, causing considerable damage not only to the skin itself but to underlying structures. Long-neglected cases around the eyes and ears have unfortunately resulted in loss of those organs. At the very least, from a cosmetic standpoint, the longer the destruction is allowed to continue, the worse the resulting permanent scarring.

There are several different varieties of basal cell cancer. The most common typically appears in its early stages as a shiny, pearly, pimple-like bump on your skin. In the later stages of basal cell cancer untreated cases, crusting, ulceration, and bleeding can occur.

Treatment: A biopsy is required for diagnosis of basal cell carcinoma, and the choice of treatments may be one of the several methods discussed earlier. In general, my first choice of therapy is curettage and electrosurgery. The procedure is quick and the healing is usually excellent. For recurrent lesions, Moh's Chemosurgery is unquestionably the preferred treatment method. If for some reason the Moh's method is not feasible, I generally refer such a patient for radiotherapy.

Squamous Cell Carcinoma

Squamous cell skin cancers are the second most common form of skin cancer in white people, affecting from eighty to one hundred thousand people annually. In general, squamous cell carcinomas that arise as a result of excessive sun damage are no more serious or potentially life-threatening than most basal cell skin cancers. Nonetheless, squamous cell carcinoma, like basal cell cancers, can also be quite locally destructive and disfiguring if neglected.

Squamous cell cancers that arise, however, in areas of chronic irritation, scarring, or prior X-ray exposure may be quite serious and potentially life-threatening. Such cancers may metastasize to other organs of the body through the bloodstream. Serious forms of squamous cell skin cancer are responsible for approximately fifteen hundred to two thousand deaths per year.

Squamous cell skin carcinomas usually appear as pink or reddish, opaque growths. They can also appear wart-like and can ulcerate in the center. Sometimes they can increase so significantly in size as to appear like large mushroom-like growths with central crusting and ulceration.

Treatment: The diagnosis and treatment alternatives for sun-damage-related squamous cell carcinomas are identical to those used for treating basal cell carcinomas. For the more serious squamous cell malignancies, wide surgical excision is usually performed first. The patient is then usually referred for consultation and further care and follow-up to an oncologist (cancer care specialist).

Malignant Melanoma

Malignant melanoma is the leading cause of death from skin cancer, accounting for 74 percent of all skin cancer deaths. The death rate from melanoma is increasing at an alarming rate, faster than any other cancer except lung cancer. In the past year, over twenty-two thousand people were discovered to have malignant melanoma and nearly six thousand died of it. It is predicted that by the year 2000, one in every 100 people in the United States will develop a malignant melanoma.

Certain individuals are at higher risk of developing malignant melanoma. As I mentioned earlier, people with melanoma precursor lesions, such as large congenital moles, dysplastic nevi, or Hutchinson's melanotic freckle, are at higher risk. In addition, fair-eyed, fair-complected persons, people who live in sunbelt or equatorial regions, those who have had episodes of severe sunburn, particularly during childhood and adolescence, and individuals who had numerous moles during childhood, are also at higher risk.

Malignant melanoma lesions may be flat or elevated, have irregular borders and outlines, exhibit multiple shades of dark brown, red, white, blue, or black, and may exhibit "spitting" out of their pigment beyond the original confines of the mole themselves into the surrounding normal skin.

Treatment: If a malignant melanoma is suspected, your dermatologist will probably perform an excisional biopsy if possible. If this is not feasible for some reason, an incisional biopsy will be performed. After the diagnosis is established, the pathologist will be able to provide some information about the overall prognosis. Simply stated, the more deeply the melanoma is found to extend into the skin, the potentially more serious the eventual outcome.

After melanoma is diagnosed, a wide surgical excision of the tumor is then performed. A certain amount of surrounding, normal-appearing skin is purposefully removed, as well, to insure that the entire melanoma is encased within the excised tissue. In other words, by taking out a little extra skin, the surgeon is trying to make sure every last bit of the melanoma is out.

It the melanoma is caught early and the lesion is not deep, surgical removal is curative 97 percent of the time. If the melanoma is deep at the time it is first diagnosed, the individual will usually need to be referred after surgery to an oncologist for follow-up and further care.

I must emphasize that far and away the best therapy for malignant melanoma remains prevention. Since the outcome of melanoma is heavily dependent upon its early recognition, the identification and removal of precancerous lesions, and the surgical removal of melanomas while they are still only superficially located in the skin, *can* be lifesaving. And if this chapter has made some of you sit up and take notice of any possibly troublesome growths on your face and body that you have been ignoring up to now, *Saving Face* may just have helped you save your life.

18

*What's New or
on the Horizon*

Research into new medical and surgical therapies for the skin is constant. New discoveries are being made at an awe-inspiring pace and older medications and treatments are continually being replaced or improved. Unfortunately, not everything new stands the test of time, and new drugs or procedures are frequently the subjects of heated controversies.

The purpose of this final chapter is not to present the controversies existing on the frontiers of science and technology but to give you some idea of new and encouraging therapeutic developments that I find personally exciting and that may have a direct effect on facial skin therapy in the not-too-distant-future. The potpourri in this chapter is by no means a complete listing of all that is new or on the horizon; that simply isn't realistic. The pace of science and technology today is too quick, and a complete list would fill *many* books.

I have chosen to include in this chapter discussions of six new or on-the-horizon developments in skin care therapy: (1) the carbon dioxide laser and some of its practical uses; (2) ZYPLAST collagen, a recently introduced form of injectable collagen; (3) FIBREL foam, a newly developed, non-collagen, non-silicone-containing fibrin foam injectable for scar and wrinkle treatment; (4) the expanding use of nitrous oxide ("laughing gas" sedation) in office-based skin surgery; (5) permanent microsurgical pigmentation, an increasingly popular technique for creating permanent eyeliners; and (6) some new drugs and some new uses for older drugs.

CARBON DIOXIDE LASER

In Chapter 13, I discussed the use of the argon laser to treat port wine stains of the face and neck. Now the carbon dioxide laser is gradually finding its way into more and more offices. It is estimated that by 1990 approximately 60 percent of all dermatologists will be using lasers to treat a wide variety of diseases. While the shorter wavelength light emitted by the argon laser is selectively absorbed by hemoglobin and melanin, the longer wavelength light emitted by the carbon dioxide laser is selectively absorbed by water. As a result, the carbon dioxide laser rapidly heats water in the tissue being treated to the boiling point, evaporating it. The carbon dioxide laser is able to evaporate unwanted tissue in a path narrower than one-twentieth of an inch.

While the jury is not yet in on the overall place of the carbon dioxide laser in skin surgery, good results have been reported in the treatment of various kinds of warts, which in some cases had not responded to repeated treatments with other chemical and surgical methods. One potential advantage of carbon dioxide laser therapy over more conventional wart removal treatments is that the operative site is sterilized by the laser beam because the wart virus particles are themselves vaporized. Theoretically, vaporizing the virus particles so that they are unable to contaminate areas adjacent to the surgical wound should decrease the chances of the wart recurring. Deep wounds have been found to heal nicely after carbon dioxide laser surgery.

The carbon dioxide laser has also been reportedly successful in removing keloid scars, reducing bulbous (rhinophyma) noses, smoothing certain kinds of acne scarring, removing tattoos, and vaporizing certain forms of skin cancer. The carbon dioxide laser possesses the additional advantage of sealing blood vessels as it cuts. This can be particularly useful for minimizing blood loss in patients with high blood pressure who cannot be given epinephrine along with the anesthetic (Epinephrine raises blood pressure.) For the same reason, it is advantageous for treating people who have abnormal bleeding tendencies, such as hemophiliacs, or people who are taking blood-thinning drugs, such as COUMADIN.

The most common complications of carbon dioxide laser surgery are the formation of "proud flesh" scars and mottled or darkened skin pigmentation. However, these have been observed in only a few patients. Only time and continued investigation of the possible uses and potential benefits of the carbon dioxide laser will determine its ultimate place in our surgical armamentarium.

ZYPLAST

Very recently, the Collagen Corporation, the developers of ZYDERM injectable collagen, introduced ZYPLAST collagen, a new form of injectable collagen. The collagen fibers in ZYPLAST collagen, unlike those in ZYDERM collagen, have been linked in such a way as to minimize their shrinkage after injection. Unlike ZYDERM collagen, which is meant to be injected more superficially into the dermis, ZYPLAST collagen is intended for injection subdermally (i.e., more deeply, below the dermis).

ZYPLAST collagen was not developed as a substitute for ZYDERM collagen. Each has its own uses. Since, by design, little implant shrinkage occurs following its placement in the skin, ZYPLAST collagen is being used in situations where ZYDERM collagen has not been found particularly useful or only partially successful. It is largely recommended for correcting subdermal defects (i.e., defects deeper than those that the more shrinkable ZYDERM collagen are ordinarily unable to adequately correct). ZYPLAST collagen is being used to elevate sunken cheeks or to create the appearance of "higher cheekbones." It is also being used, for example, to smooth out skin contour irregularities that may form around the nose after rhinoplasty; to elevate extremely deep wrinkle lines; to puff out particularly deep scars; and to add body to what would otherwise be thin and sunken-appearing burn scar and skin graft sites. ZYPLAST collagen is also being tested for improving some types of postsurgical scarring, such as those that can sometimes result from extensive Moh's Chemosurgery.

Since ZYPLAST collagen has only recently been granted FDA approval, it has not yet been used nearly as extensively as ZYDERM collagen. To date, few side effects have been observed in the nearly one thousand people who have so far been treated with it. More extensive testing and experience are needed to see whether ZYPLAST collagen, like its sibling ZYDERM collagen, will survive the test of time.

FIBREL (INJECTABLE
FIBRIN FOAM)

FIBREL foam, a new, noncollagen, non-silicone-containing injectable product for the treatment of various kinds of depressed scars, has recently been tested in twenty-five centers throughout the country. Still under intense investigation, FIBREL foam has not yet been granted Food and Drug Administration approval for widespread use. Initial reports have claimed that FIBREL foam and ZYDERM injectable collagen are equally effective for the correction of depressed scars.

On the other hand, FIBREL foam is claimed to be less allergenic than ZYDERM collagen, and may result in longer lasting corrections. In laboratory animals, some investigators found that FIBREL foam caused less inflammation at injection sites and was responsible for more new collagen deposition than ZYDERM collagen.

The technique for injecting FIBREL foam is identical to that of ZYDERM collagen. Just as with ZYDERM collagen, temporary redness, black and blue marks, swelling, and a mild burning or stinging sensation may occur at the injection sites. FIBREL foam's treatment protocol is also like that of ZYDERM collagen: a small test dose is placed in the forearm one month prior to initiating actual therapy and subsequent treatments are administered at two- to four-week intervals.

FIBREL foam consists of three major components: gelatin, a chemical called aminocaproic acid, and the patient's own blood plasma. It is believed to work as follows. First, the injection of FIBREL foam is believed to result in mild tissue injury at the injection site. In response to this injury, the body begins producing new collagen. The injected plasma supports the new collagen formation by providing many necessary blood plasma factors. Finally, the gelatin acts both to trap and hold together all the important ingredients for new collagen formation. It also acts as a template for the laying down of the new collagen. Thus far, the results with FIBREL in the treatment of acne, chicken pox, and traumatic scars have been very encouraging. If further testing bears out these initial findings, FIBREL foam may prove to be a safe and effective alternative to ZYDERM collagen therapy for the treatment of depressed scars and wrinkles.

NITROUS OXIDE ANALGESIA
(CONSCIOUS SEDATION)

As the medical editor of the *Journal of the American Analgesia Society*, a professional journal specifically devoted to exploring methods for reducing anxiety and pain during office surgery, I have been particularly involved in exploring the uses of nitrous oxide in cosmetic and dermatologic office surgery. I first became interested in this subject several years ago, when, about to undergo some routine office surgery, a patient asked me why I wasn't sedating her with "gas" like her dentist did.

The simple truth is that, unfortunately, the administration of nitrous oxide analgesia is simply not taught, either in American medical schools or most residency training programs. The historical reasons for that omission are still unclear to me today. Nevertheless, my patient had given me a great idea, and within a year I had gotten the necessary training needed to administer nitrous oxide gas (See Chapter 12).

Physiologists have known of the effects of nitrous oxide for nearly a century and a half. For years nitrous oxide has been routinely used by many dentists for pain control. Many of you may even be somewhat familiar with it. The unfortunate fact is that for many years nitrous oxide has largely remained within the exclusive province of dental surgery.

It has been only during the past couple of years that nitrous oxide analgesia for pain and anxiety alleviation has begun to be used for nondental surgery, particularly cosmetic and dermatologic office surgery. However, most cosmetic surgeons wishing to learn more about nitrous oxide must still obtain their classroom and hands-on training through courses given periodically throughout the country by the various regional dental societies. Happily, this is now beginning to change.

As more and more surgical procedures are shifted from the hospital setting to the office setting, I believe we will see a rapidly expanding interest in the use of nitrous oxide, as well as other forms of analgesia and sedation by many office-based dermatologic and cosmetic surgeons. As a result, there will no doubt be an increase in medical courses and seminars devoted to these subjects. While nitrous oxide analgesia is not for everyone, unquestionably, most routine office-based procedures, running the gamut from multiple collagen injections, chemical peels, acne surgery, skin cancer surgery, etc., can be made less disconcerting and less uncomfortable with the use of "sweet air."

Ask your doctor about it. There is no reason for needless suffering.

PERMANENT
MICROPIGMENTATION
SURGERY

Permanent micropigmentation surgery, a technique for creating a permanent eyeliner, has been used by a handful of ophthalmic plastic surgeons for a few years. Recently, it has become the subject of increasing interest by a growing number of plastic and dermatologic cosmetic surgeons. However, at the present time, few of them actually perform the technique. This technique for creating a "permanent eyeliner" is, in some respects, similar to tattooing. Unlike tattooing, however, the pigment is placed very superficially in the eyelid skin, rather than deeply.

A number of people can be benefited by this procedure. Obviously those who dislike the daily routine of applying eye cosmetics would benefit from the convenience of having an attractive eyeliner permanently "tattooed" in place. Those who are allergic to commercial eyeliner cosmetics may find microsurgical pigmentation a welcome alternative. In addition, individuals who wear extended-wear contact lenses and are concerned about the risk of corneal abrasions from particles of cosmetic eyeliners embedding under the lenses, could also benefit from microsurgical pigmentation. Persons suffering from disabling arthritis who have lost the dexterity to apply eye makeup make ideal candidates for permanent eyeliner surgery.

Eyebrow reconstruction and enhancement, and repigmentation of depigmented, burned, scarred, or hairless areas of the skin are some additional uses of permanent microsurgical pigmentation that are currently being explored.

The *raison d'être* for its initial development, namely *permanence*, remains the major drawback to the permanent microsurgical pigmentation. So before you opt for having permanent eyeliner surgery, bear in mind the following. As you get older or fashions change, you may find that the permanent style and shades of eyeliner you originally chose are no longer appropriate for you. Once you do it, you're stuck with it!

Permanent eyeliner is applied with an electrical instrument. A portable handpiece with needles for superficially penetrating the eyelid skin at the base of the lashes is used to place iron oxide pigment into the eyelid skin. Iron oxide seldom causes allergy. (India ink and other potentially harmful dyes used in regular tattooing are not used in microsurgical eyelining.) The intensity of color shading depends upon the application time and the use of lighteners. The longer the application time, the deeper the intensity. The procedure takes about thirty minutes to perform.

Talc, which is used by some manufacturers as a lightening agent for the eyeliner pigment, is a known cause of a special type of deep allergic inflammation of the skin, called a *granuloma*. So far, granuloma formation has not been observed in the over five hundred eyelining procedures that have been performed. However, granuloma development typically requires about five years to manifest itself. For this reason, one manufacturer has already replaced talc with titanium oxide, a substance not known to cause granulomas.

SOME NEW DRUGS
AND SOME NEW USES
FOR OLD DRUGS

In this final section I would like to say a few words about several important medications you will no doubt be hearing a good deal more about in the near future: *etretinate, viprostil, spriro-nolactone,* and *isotretinoin.* Etretinate and viprostil are new drugs. Spironolactone is a potassium-sparing diuretic (water-pill) that has been in use for a number of years, and isotretinoin

(ACCUTANE capsules), discussed in Chapter 15, is an extremely potent oral anti-cystic acne medication.

Etretinate (Tigason), a chemical relative of ACCUTANE capsules, is also an oral, synthetic vitamin A derivative. It has been extensively tested in Europe on patients with psoriasis who have not responded well to intensive conventional anti-psoriasis therapies, and impressive results have been obtained in patients with severe forms of psoriasis.

Etretinate does share many of the same side effects as ACCU-TANE capsules. However, it is known to persist considerably longer in the body than ACCUTANE capsules after therapy has been discontinued. There also seems to be a higher risk of fetal birth defects, possibly due to this longer "washout" period.

Preliminary studies of etretinate in psoriasis treatment are currently taking place in the United States. People taking it require careful physician-monitoring. Should these investigations bear out the encouraging promise of the European findings, it is likely that the FDA will approve etretinate for use here in the not-too-distant future.

Viprostol is an anti-high-blood pressure medicine that recently received a great deal of press coverage for its potential hair restoring ability when topically applied. Not unexpectedly, the limited success of topically applied minoxidil has spurred a search for other potentially topically applied antihypertensive medications that might be even more effective for stimulating hair regrowth than minoxidil. Little more can be said about viprostol at this time since clinical trials of this drug have just begun. Several years and much testing will be required before any definite statements about its efficacy can be made. But it does mean that for those of you suffering from a hair loss problem, there is one more reason to be hopeful.

Spironolactone, long used as an effective potassium-sparing water pill, has preliminarily been found to have a potential role in the treatment of a completely unrelated condition—severe acne vulgaris. As you already know, male hormones (androgens) in women and men play a significant role in acne formation and increased oil gland secretion. Spironolactone has been found to block the action of the male hormone, and it is this effect that is considered responsible for its beneficial role in severe acne. Further testing of spironolactone is required in larger numbers of patients before this drug can be recommended and routinely prescribed. A further encouraging note: few side effects were noted in the initial studies of spironolactone for the treatment of severe acne.

Finally, isotretinoin (ACCUTANE capsules) is being actively tested for a role that takes it far afield from its successful use in the treatment of severe cystic acne vulgaris—the prevention of skin cancers. Laboratory studies have suggested that isotretinoin may slow or prevent malignant transformation. To test this out, large scale studies in humans are under way, but the results of these studies will not be available for another few years. It is hoped that isotretinoin, or perhaps some other chemical relative of it with fewer potential side effects, may be able to prevent the formation of the numerous sun-related precancers and skin cancers that plague so many of us. Researchers are also looking to see whether isotretinoin in appropriate doses can reverse the formation of malignant skin growths once they have fully formed. As you may well imagine, an effective oral drug for the prevention and therapy of skin malignancies would make a more-than-welcome alternative to our present surgical methods. Given the widespread nature of the skin cancer problem, finding a safe and convenient oral drug is obviously of enormous health and cosmetic importance, and would take us one giant step closer to truly saving face.

Index